Cardiac Rehabilitation

Cardiac Rehabilitation

A Workbook for use with Group Programmes

Julian Bath

Gail Bohin

Christine Jones

Eve Scarle

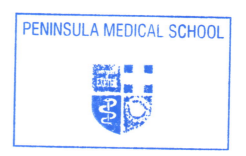

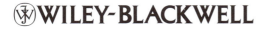

A John Wiley & Sons, Ltd., Publication

This edition first published 2009

© 2009 John Wiley & Sons Ltd.

Wiley-Blackwell is an imprint of John Wiley & Sons, formed by the merger of Wiley's global Scientific, Technical, and Medical business with Blackwell Publishing.

Registered Office

John Wiley & Sons Ltd, The Atrium, Southern Gate, Chichester, West Sussex, PO19 8SQ, UK

Editorial Offices

The Atrium, Southern Gate, Chichester, West Sussex, PO19 8SQ, UK

9600 Garsington Road, Oxford, OX4 2DQ, UK

350 Main Street, Malden, MA 02148-5020, USA

For details of our global editorial offices, for customer services, and for information about how to apply for permission to reuse the copyright material in this book please see our website at www.wiley.com/wiley-blackwell.

The right of the authors to be identified as the author of this work has been asserted in accordance with the Copyright, Designs and Patents Act 1988.

Wiley also publishes its books in a variety of electronic formats. Some content that appears in print may not be available in electronic books.

Designations used by companies to distinguish their products are often claimed as trademarks. All brand names and product names used in this book are trade names, service marks, trademarks or registered trademarks of their respective owners. The publisher is not associated with any product or vendor mentioned in this book.

This publication is designed to provide accurate and authoritative information in regard to the subject matter covered. It is sold on the understanding that the publisher is not engaged in rendering professional services. If professional advice or other expert assistance is required, the services of a competent professional should be sought.

Library of Congress Cataloging-in-Publication Data

Cardiac rehabilitation: a workbook for use with group programmes/Julian Bath . . . [et al.].
    p.; cm.
  Includes bibliographical references and index.
  ISBN 978-0-470-51872-4
  1. Heart—Diseases—Patients—Rehabilitation. I. Bath, Julian.
  [DNLM: 1. Cardiovascular Diseases—rehabilitation—Great Britain. 2. Exercise
Therapy—methods–Great Britain. 3. Group Processes—Great Britain. 4. Health Behavior—Great Britain.
5. Risk Reduction Behavior—Great Britain. WG 166 C26472 2010]
  RC682.C368 2010
  616.1'203–dc22

                                                                       2009029987

A catalogue record for this book is available from the British Library.

Set in 12/13.5 Times by Thomson Digital

Printed and bound in Singapore by Fabulous Pte Ltd

1 2009

Contents

Abbreviations Used in This Book

AACVPR	American Association of Cardiovascular and Pulmonary Rehabilitation
ACPICR	Association of Chartered Physiotherapists in Cardiac Rehabilitation
ACS	acute coronary syndrome
AR	active recovery
BACR	British Association for Cardiac Rehabilitation
BMI	body mass index
CABG	coronary artery bypass graft
CHD	coronary heart disease
CHF	chronic heart failure
CPD	continuing professional development
CR	cardiac rehabilitation
CV	cardiovascular
ECG	electro-cardiogram
GTN	glyceryl trinitrate
HRR	heart rate reserve
ICD	implantable cardioverter defibrillators
IPDR	individual performance and development review
IPQ	Illness Perception Questionnaire
MDT	multidisciplinary team
MHR	maximum heart rate
MI	myocardial infarction
NACR	National Audit for Cardiac Rehabilitation
NSF	National Service Framework
PCI	percutaneous coronary intervention
PDP	personal development plan
RHR	resting heart rate
RPE	Rate of Perceived Exertion (also known as Modified BORG Scale)
SRM	self-regulatory model
WHO	World Health Organization

About the Authors

Julian Bath is a Consultant Health Psychologist based at Gloucestershire Royal Hospital with ten years' experience of working in cardiac rehabilitation in Gloucestershire. He also has experience of working in renal, diabetes and rheumatology services. He has a wide range of knowledge, skills and experience in health psychology, including consultancy work, published book chapters and research papers and teaching/training of health professionals and students to doctoral level.

Gail Bohin is a Clinical Psychologist with Gloucestershire Cardiac Rehabilitation Service. In addition to contributing to the multidisciplinary rehabilitation group programme she also works individually with cardiac patients. Since completing her doctoral training in 1999, she has worked with a variety of patient populations in both physical and mental health and primary and secondary care. These include primary care psychology for working-age adults, oncology, palliative care, stroke, older adults and renal care.

Christine Jones is a Cardiac Rehabilitation Specialist Nurse with nearly 20 years' experience of working with cardiac patients, including five years in her current post in Gloucestershire. In addition to delivering cardiac rehabilitation Christine is link nurse for patients with implantable cardioverter defibrillators and has a special interest in arrhythmias.

Eve Scarle has worked as a physiotherapist for the past seven years, five of which have been spent working in cardiac rehabilitation. She has recently taken up a post as Lecturer in Sport and Physical Activity at the University of Gloucestershire. Eve has a keen interest in exercise for referred populations and has been instrumental in setting up a cardiovascular and GP exercise referral scheme for the university. She also has a background in working in gyms and health clubs, teaching exercise to music and gym instruction.

Preface

The principal aim of this book is simple: to provide a practical framework for a multidisciplinary team to deliver a cardiac rehabilitation (CR) group programme. Cardiac rehabilitation programmes have historically been set up in many different formats, from exercise-only programmes through to multidisciplinary team programmes that can involve four or more different health professionals. These programmes have also managed a variety of different conditions, from coronary heart disease (CHD) through to patients with valve conditions and implantable cardioverter defibrillators (ICDs). This book describes the management of coronary heart disease patients through the cardiac rehabilitation group programme in Gloucestershire (although it would be quite possible to adapt the programme's content for use in managing other cardiac patient populations). The content is presented in a way that should enable a team of trained staff, such as cardiac nurses, exercise professionals, psychologists and dieticians, to understand and deliver a seven-week cardiac rehabilitation programme.

A secondary aim of the book is to provide a useful introduction to the topic of cardiac rehabilitation. We will therefore give a brief history of the development of cardiac rehabilitation in the UK and discuss evidence for its role in the management of coronary heart disease. The National Service Framework for Coronary Heart Disease, published in March 2000, set out the government's intention, over 10 years, to improve the care of patients with CHD, and described a number of standards for the improved prevention, diagnosis, treatment and rehabilitation of individuals with CHD. The standard for cardiac rehabilitation (Chapter 7) states that, prior to leaving hospital, individuals suffering from CHD should be invited to participate in a multidisciplinary programme of secondary prevention and cardiac rehabilitation (Department of Health, 2000). The aim of such a programme is to reduce the risk of subsequent cardiac problems and to promote the return to a full and normal life. However, the provision of cardiac rehabilitation varies widely across the UK, from "exercise-only" programmes to "comprehensive" programmes that are delivered by multidisciplinary teams of health professionals and include exercise training, behavioural change approaches, education and psychological support. Who delivers this comprehensive, multidisciplinary CR can also vary widely across the UK, with nurses, doctors, psychologists, physiotherapists, exercise specialists, occupational therapists and dieticians all potentially involved. Furthermore, service delivery models tend to vary from county to county, and currently there is no accepted "manual" for use in the delivery of cardiac rehabilitation in the UK. One reason why some CR programmes lack the behavioural change and educational aspects found in comprehensive CR programmes is the complex and time-consuming nature of planning and preparing such a programme. One of the aims of this book is to minimise the planning and preparation time involved in setting up and delivering a CR programme and to present the relevant information and techniques in a way that can be used confidently by a variety of different health professionals.

The bulk of the book is made up of the session plans for the seven weeks over which the cardiac rehabilitation programme is run in Gloucestershire. The "Gloucestershire Model" of CR (described in more detail in Chapter 2) is one of the many ways in which CR group programmes are delivered in the UK, and as such it is not intended that this model should be seen as definitive. However, it is hoped that the session plans which describe the programme will be useful to any health professional involved in setting up a CR programme, whichever model is being used. The challenge has been to present the material in an accessible manner with sufficient detail to enable different multidisciplinary team professionals to deliver the appropriate sessions. The exercise programme could potentially be delivered as a series of stand-alone sessions, but is fully integrated into the educational and behavioural change part of the "comprehensive" programme through the concepts of pacing, goal-setting and "making changes". Similarly the education/behavioural change aspects of the programme are presented in such a way that they could be used as an adjunct to an existing exercise programme.

In addition to the session plans, the introductory chapters briefly describe the history of cardiac rehabilitation in the UK, review the important evidence for the efficacy of CR, outline the CR programme in Gloucestershire (and how to prepare for such a programme) and discuss the practical application of exercise in a cardiac rehabilitation programme. The important psychological theory that underpins the programme is also discussed.

The session plan material outlined in this book arose from work that has been carried out in cardiac rehabilitation in Gloucestershire over the past 16 years. The multidisciplinary CR group programme in Gloucestershire has developed and changed considerably over the past decade and a half (as new evidence has emerged), and the supporting literature that has been given to patients has changed along with the programme. Although handouts have been given to patients attending the CR programme over the years, literature which enables new staff coming into cardiac rehabilitation to learn how to deliver the group programme has been limited. The will to put together a "manual" for the cardiac rehabilitation group programmes in Gloucestershire has been evident for many years, but the resources have not previously been available to enable its production. The time-limited resources available to most NHS cardiac rehabilitation programmes make it very difficult to develop a training manual for

CR, and in turn without such a tool it is sometimes difficult for individuals who are setting up and running new programmes to be sure of their efficacy. It is hoped that this book will help to fill the gap, providing a manual for the delivery of cardiac rehabilitation group programmes by a multidisciplinary team. In addition it is hoped that it will provide a useful introduction to cardiac rehabilitation for trainees and students of health and clinical psychology as well as physiotherapy, nursing, occupational therapy and medical staff.

A large number of health professionals have been involved in the cardiac rehabilitation programme in Gloucestershire over the past 16 years, and many of them have helped to shape the programme into the format in which it exists today and which we describe in this book. One individual, Dr Louise Earll, has been central to this process. It was Dr Earll who initially set up the programme and who continued to have a direct input into CR in Gloucestershire until 2005. Suffice it to say that if Dr Earll had not been involved in cardiac rehabilitation then this book would not have been written. Many thanks are due to Dr Earll for her influence and legacy. Thanks are due to the other health professionals who have actively informed our practice and supported our work, namely Professor Marie Johnston, Professor Bob Lewin, Professor Susan Michie, Dr Karen Rodham, Dr Mark Peterson and Dr David Lyndsay. Thanks should also be given to Julia Harrison, Alison Anderson, Jan Harding, Ann McArley (and the dietetics team) and Maggie Gallacher, past and present members of the Gloucestershire CR team, who have all been instrumental in shaping the programme over the past decade and more.

Chapter 1
Multidisciplinary Cardiac Rehabilitation

This introductory chapter will briefly describe the evidence for the use of cardiac rehabilitation (CR) in the management of coronary heart disease and how this evidence has influenced the shift from exercise-only programmes to the comprehensive multidisciplinary CR programmes that are prominent in the UK today.

Background

By 2005 coronary heart disease (CHD) had become the leading cause of death in the UK, killing more than 110,000 people each year in England alone (Department of Health, 2005). Furthermore, approximately 275,000 people experienced a myocardial infarction (MI), or heart attack, each year, with a further 1.4 million people suffering from angina (Department of Health, 2005). Currently coronary heart disease accounts for approximately one in five deaths in men and one in six deaths in women (British Heart Foundation, 2008). The National Service Framework (NSF) for Coronary Heart Disease, published in March 2000, set out the government's intention to improve the care of patients with CHD over a 10-year period (Department of Health, 2000). The NSF for CHD set out 12 standards for the improved prevention, diagnosis, treatment and rehabilitation of people with coronary heart disease and aimed to secure fair access to high-quality services. One such service is cardiac rehabilitation, and chapter 7 of the NSF, "Cardiac Rehabilitation", outlined a national standard (Standard Twelve) for the rehabilitation of patients with CHD:

> NHS trusts should put in place agreed protocols/systems of care so that, prior to leaving hospital, people admitted to hospital suffering from coronary heart disease have been invited to participate in a multidisciplinary programme of secondary prevention and cardiac rehabilitation. The aim of the programme will be to reduce their risk of subsequent cardiac problems and to promote their return to a full and normal life.
>
> (Department of Health, 2000)

Cardiac Rehabilitation

In 1993 cardiac rehabilitation was defined by the World Health Organization (WHO) as:

> the sum of activities required to influence favourably the underlying cause of the disease, as well as the best possible, physical, mental and social conditions, so that they [people] may, by their own efforts preserve or resume when lost, as normal a place as possible in the community. Rehabilitation cannot be regarded as an isolated form or stage of therapy but must be integrated within secondary prevention services of which it forms only one facet.
>
> (World Health Organization, 1993)

The stated aim of the WHO definition of cardiac rehabilitation that it must "be integrated within secondary prevention services" has been accepted as the norm for CR services today. The drive towards helping individuals to return to "their former way of life" facilitated the rise of multidisciplinary cardiac rehabilitation (Dusseldorp et al., 1999). Multidisciplinary CR involves using a team of nurses, exercise specialists, psychologists, dieticians and other health professionals to bring together medical treatment, education, counselling, exercise training, risk-factor modification and secondary prevention (Thompson and De Bono, 1999). The definition of cardiac rehabilitation in the NSF for CHD acknowledges these factors and updates the earlier WHO definition, incorporating the concepts of lifestyle change and individual confidence:

> To enable people to achieve the lifestyle changes that they want to make and to regain their confidence so that they can enjoy the best possible physical, mental and emotional health and so return to as full and as normal a life as possible.
>
> (Department of Health, 2000)

Does Cardiac Rehabilitation Work?

Meta-analyses of the effectiveness of cardiac rehabilitation programmes in the late 1980s showed that CR was associated with a reduction in both cardiac and all-cause mortality (O'Connor et al., 1989; Oldridge et al, 1988). A decade later, a University of York NHS Centre for Reviews and Dissemination report (1998) suggested that cardiac rehabilitation could "promote recovery, enable patients to achieve and maintain better health, and reduce risk of death in people with heart disease". As the efficacy of CR became evident in the 1990s, the number of CR programmes across the country multiplied and the importance of increasing attendance at them became a priority. A randomised controlled trial by Wyer et al. (2001) in Gloucestershire showed that simple, cost-effective and theory-driven interventions (in this case an invitation letter based on a health behaviour change model: the Theory of Planned Behaviour) could increase attendance at cardiac rehabilitation, enabling more patients to experience its perceived benefits. However, UK statistics at this time suggested that only approximately 23 per cent of all MI patients were enrolling on CR, with a slightly higher figure for those undergoing a coronary artery bypass graft (CABG), "participation rates being between 33% and 56%" (Bethell et al., 2001). Adherence to CR programmes was also proving problematic, with only a third of patients continuing to participate in an exercise programme six months after completing their group sessions (Daly et al., 2002). Consistent findings on the barriers to participating in cardiac rehabilitation included lack of physician referral, being female, being older, of lower educational status, having poor functional capacity and having had an angioplasty as opposed to CABG (Daly et al., 2002; Turner et al., 2002).

Cardiac rehabilitation was producing financial savings through a reduction in readmission rates to hospital and improvements in re-employment (Pell, 1997). However, as secondary care programmes became more comprehensive, particularly with the widespread prescription of statins and other cardiac medication, the evidence for the effectiveness of CR began to be questioned. West, in 2002, argued that there was little evidence for the current efficacy of cardiac rehabilitation following acute MI, as there had been few recent trials. He suggested that the historic trials from the 1980s may have lost relevance because of the changing methods of treatment in coronary care units. In particular, he argued that the prescription of medication and early use of thrombolytics, or "clot-busting" medication (which if given in the first few hours after a myocardial infarction can limit damage to the heart), led to the efficacy of CR being diminished. A multicentre randomised controlled trial in 14 hospitals of patients attending "comprehensive" CR, as opposed to "usual care", found no differences in mortality, further cardiac events, quality of life, anxiety or depression (West, 2002). Minor differences in outcome were evident in CR patients taking fewer long-acting nitrates and in positive uptake of exercise. Patients also reported that they found their CR programmes to be generally beneficial.

Recent Evidence for the Efficacy of Cardiac Rehabilitation

A meta-analysis by Clark et al. (2005) challenged West's argument for the potentially ineffectual nature of CR following the recent advances in secondary prevention medication. In a review of 63 randomised controlled trials, including exercise-only CR, comprehensive CR and educational (non-exercise)

CR from 1966 to 2004, Clark found that CR reduced mortality by 47 per cent at two-year follow-up, decreased subsequent MI by 17 per cent over a median follow-up of 12 months and improved functional quality of life (Clark et al., 2005). Furthermore, Clark found that the mortality benefit did not differ significantly between the older trials from the 1980s that reported a decrease in mortality following CR, and the more recent trials. This puts into doubt the argument that secondary prevention medication had negated the impact of CR programmes. Although benefits did not differ between the three types of CR that were analysed in this study, Clark suggests that this kind of review does not allow us to "determine the incremental benefits of the various components of each intervention" (Clark et al., 2005) and therefore does not allow us to judge which aspects of CR are the important or "active" ingredients. Clark looked at three different types of CR in his meta-analysis: those programmes that incorporated education and counselling about coronary risk factors with a supervised education programme; those programmes that included risk-factor education or counselling but no exercise component; and those programmes that consisted solely of a structured exercise programme (Clark et al., 2005). However, Clark recognises a variety of different types, and a range of frequency and intensity, in the educational, counselling and exercise aspects of the CR programmes within his study.

A more recent meta-analysis by Linden (Linden et al., 2007) looked at the outcomes of studies where there was a psychological intervention involved in the CR programme. Linden found that across 23 studies, having a "clearly identifiable, distinct psychological treatment" as part of the patient's care led to a 27 per cent reduction in mortality for at least the first two years compared with normal care, and a reduced event reoccurrence at long-term follow-up. However these results only applied to men, with women not gaining the mortality benefits. This has led to a call for more research looking at gender outcomes in CR. It has also reinforced the importance of having multidisciplinary teams involved in delivering "comprehensive" cardiac rehabilitation.

Comprehensive Cardiac Rehabilitation

Dalal et al. (2004), describing the developments in CR at that time, outlined the distinction between "exercise only" and "comprehensive" cardiac rehabilitation. Comprehensive cardiac rehabilitation is described as including exercise training, behavioural change approaches, education and psychological support. In comprehensive CR, long-term maintenance of physical activity and lifestyle change is "coupled with structured follow up to tackle secondary prevention risk factors" (Dalal et al., 2004). However, the extensive surveys of cardiac rehabilitation provision in the UK that have been undertaken in the last 10 years (Bethell et al., 2001, 2007; Brodie et al., 2006; Lewin et al., 1998) have shown wide variance in how, by whom and to whom this "comprehensive" cardiac rehabilitation is delivered. Bethell found that, of the 236 CR centres that provided survey data, 194 had nurse involvement in their programmes, compared to only 37 programmes that had a psychologist involved in delivering cardiac rehabilitation (Bethell et al., 2001). An earlier study by Lewin et al. (1998) found that, although 70 per cent of CR programmes in their survey reported having five or more health-care professions represented in their CR teams, in only a small number of these teams did physicians (16 per cent), a psychologist (9 per cent) or a health promotion officer (6 per cent) give talks to patients or take any other part in the CR programme. Brodie et al. (2006), in a random sample survey of 28 CR programmes across England, reported that co-ordinators of the services considered lack of psychologists to be the greatest deficiency in the service (57 per cent) followed by lack of physiotherapists (43 per cent). These data become even more important when considering the findings of the meta-analysis by Linden et al. (2007), which showed mortality benefits in men, at two years post-cardiac event, when they were given a psychological treatment in addition to usual care as part of their cardiac rehabilitation. Overall the data suggest that CR in the UK can be described as multidisciplinary, but the distribution of health professionals across different CR programmes is inconsistent, ultimately affecting the quality of patient care.

Comprehensive Cardiac Rehabilitation in Gloucestershire

Comprehensive CR such as that delivered by the Gloucestershire CR team consists of a multidisciplinary team (MDT) of nurse, exercise specialist and psychologist attending each session of the seven-week programme (Cardiac Rehabilitation Gloucestershire, 2004). Access to a dietician is also provided as part of the MDT service. Health-outcome data from this programme have shown that comprehensive CR can be effective across a range of health outcomes when delivered in an integrated, multidisciplinary way (Bath et al., 2004). The conflicting health outcome data (Clark et al., 2005; West 2002), and the wide variation in the make-up of "comprehensive" CR programmes, raise the question of what are the specific ingredients that make for an effective CR programme. The findings of meta-analyses can cancel out contradictory findings where one CR service may be effective while another service is not (Michie et al., 2005). Different patient groups are often studied together in meta-analyses that consider the effectiveness of CR. So although there have been studies that have considered CABG patients alongside other patients with coronary heart disease following comprehensive CR (Engblom et al., 1992;

Seki et al., 2003; Stagmo et al., 2001; Sundin et al., 2003; Vestold Heartcare Study, 2003), most studies have considered MI patients alone. Furthermore, if certain multidisciplinary aspects of CR are missing or poorly delivered it might well be that CR then becomes less effective. Psychological and social factors in particular are often poorly assessed and addressed in CR (Lewin, 1998), despite the fact that the government recognises that tackling these areas is an important goal of cardiac rehabilitation (Department of Health, 2000). The important psychological factors involved in CR will be discussed in more detail in Chapter 2.

While certain CR programmes have three or more different health professionals attending the programme for its duration (Cardiac Rehabilitation Gloucestershire, 2004), other CR programmes that would be described as "comprehensive" may not adhere to the guidelines laid down in the NSF for CHD. Brodie et al. (2006) stated that many programmes did not meet the Scottish Intercollegiate Guideline Network for CR (SIGN, 2002), which states that there should be 6.2 full-time equivalent staff to every 500 patients. This guideline was adopted by the British Association for Cardiac Rehabilitation (BACR), the recognised national body for cardiac rehabilitation in the UK, in its Standards and Core Components for Cardiac Rehabilitation in 2007, setting minimum requirements for CR teams that include, among others, psychologists, dieticians and audit and clerical staff.

The British Association for Cardiac Rehabilitation Standards and Core Components for Cardiac Rehabilitation (2007)

In defining a set of minimum standards and core components for CR services, the BACR recognised that it would be a "big challenge for many services" to achieve them. However the organisation is aiming for a more equitable provision of CR across the UK with clearly defined core components, so that the "integrity of cardiac rehabilitation" can be protected.

The BACR outlines six standards for CR:

1. A co-ordinator who has overall responsibility for the CR service.
2. A CR core team of professionally qualified staff with appropriate skills and competencies to deliver the service.
3. A standardised assessment of individual patient needs.
4. Referral and access for the targeted patient population.
5. Registration and submission of data to the National Audit for Cardiac Rehabilitation (NACR).
6. A CR budget appropriate to meet the full service costs.

Meeting these six standards is essential for CR services to attain "full rehabilitation programme" status, and the NACR database (referred to in standard 5) will collect data from programmes and monitor their effectiveness. In combination with the six well-defined core components for cardiac rehabilitation (lifestyle; education; risk-factor management; psychosocial cardio-protective drug therapy and implantable devices; long-term management strategy), these standards make it possible to see a future whereby cardiac rehabilitation is equitable and consistently practised across the UK.

Chapter 2

The Cardiac Rehabilitation Programme in Gloucestershire

The first part of this chapter introduces the Gloucestershire cardiac rehabilitation group programme; the second part discusses some of the important issues that patients may experience following a cardiac event and some of the psychological theory that helps us to understand these issues and to plan a programme of cardiac rehabilitation.

Cardiac Rehabilitation in Gloucestershire

Based loosely on the Angina Management Programme that was running in Edinburgh at the time (Lewin et al., 1995), the Gloucestershire Cardiac Rehabilitation Service has been in existence since 1992. The current aim of the programme is to meet the needs of people with coronary heart disease in Gloucestershire who require rehabilitation following a cardiac event. The service is currently offered to patients who have experienced myocardial infarction (MI), acute coronary syndrome (ACS), a coronary artery bypass graft (CABG), or a percutaneous coronary intervention (PCI), patients who have been newly diagnosed with angina and patients with valvular heart disease. The stated purpose of the service—which mirrors the NSF for CHD aims for cardiac rehabilitation—is

> to help patients to return to as full and normal a life as possible, to regain their confidence, and to enable them to make any lifestyle changes that they wish to. This should enable them to enjoy the best physical, mental, and emotional health, and the best quality of life possible.
>
> (Department of Health, 2000)

Where the CR Service is Delivered

Cardiac rehabilitation in Gloucestershire is delivered both individually and in a group format. Patients with coronary heart disease are usually offered the CR group programme, whereas patients with valvular heart disease (or, more rarely, patients who have had a heart transplant) are offered an individual assessment and individual support from a member of the CR team. In 2008–9 there were 11 CR groups running each week across Gloucestershire over six different sites. All of these sites are in the community, with groups being held at leisure centres, GP surgeries or community centres, enabling easier patient access to the service. Findings from the Health Technology Assessment Report of 2004 (Beswick et al., 2004) estimated that 45–67 per cent of eligible patients are referred for CR nationally, with 27–41 per cent attending outpatient programmes. Local attendance rates in Gloucestershire exceed the national average (54 per cent who were referred actually attended in 2006–7). This is in part due to the wide availability of CR groups across the county.

What Does CR Look Like in Gloucestershire?

All patients in Gloucestershire who have experienced MI, acute coronary syndrome, CABG, angioplasty or newly diagnosed angina are offered a 45-minute assessment with a member of the CR team. This assessment considers patients' individual risk factors and links them to the causality and development of their coronary heart disease. Patients are also invited to attend the CR group programme at this assessment. Patients who do not wish to attend the group programme are able to access individual one-to-one support from a psychologist, cardiac nurse or physiotherapist (see below) from the CR team. The CR Service in Gloucestershire offers a seven-week group programme to people with CHD following their cardiac event. Patients attend one two-hour session per week and then two follow-up sessions at eight weeks and then eight months after the end of the seven-week programme. A multidisciplinary team consisting of a cardiac nurse, an exercise specialist and a psychologist deliver the programme. The content of the programme focuses on changing lifestyles, including exercise, diet and stress management, and is outlined in detail from Chapter 5 onwards.

Individual CR

For a variety of reasons a group programme may not be appropriate for all CR patients (for example some patients dislike group programmes, or may have issues with anxiety, depression or other health problems preventing them from attending a group programme). Patients who do not wish to, or cannot, attend a group programme can be offered an individual CR service. In this individual service patients are invited to an initial outpatient appointment with a member of the CR team. If it is not possible for a patient to attend an outpatient appointment at the hospital, a telephone appointment, or in some cases an appointment in a local GP surgery, will be offered. Depending on the reason that a patient is not able to attend the group programme, this appointment could be arranged with a psychologist, a cardiac nurse, a physiotherapist or a dietician. Onward referral is possible at this stage to the Individual CR Psychology Service.

The Individual CR Psychology Service

The NSF for CHD states that a small percentage of cardiac patients may benefit from "more formal psychological interventions such as cognitive behavioural therapy" (Department of Health, 2000). In 2003 the Individual CR Psychology Service was created in Gloucestershire, providing one-to-one sessions for CR patients, either as an alternative to or as an adjunct to the CR group programme. It offers time-limited, evidence-based psychological interventions with a clinical or health psychologist, with the aim of promoting physical and emotional recovery, by:

- Reducing distress and increasing understanding of CHD by correcting cardiac misconceptions or illness perceptions that could result in anxiety, depression or poor post-cardiac event adjustment
- Providing the time and privacy to explore issues in greater depth, using a variety of psychological techniques, including cognitive-behavioural approaches, with the aim of increasing motivation and adherence to treatment
- Offering evidence-based psychological interventions for depression, anxiety and panic disorders
- Increasing patients' confidence in their ability to manage their CHD by reinforcing the positive self-management messages of the CR group programme

Attendance at CR in Gloucestershire

In 2006–7, from a total of 1,449 CR assessments, 68 per cent of those assessed (989 people) agreed to start a CR programme. Of these, 79 per cent (778 people) actually started a programme. On average, 11 people started each CR group. Of those who started the programme, 54 per cent had a primary diagnosis of MI, while 24 per cent had experienced CABG and 21 per cent were PCI patients. Of those who did not agree to start a programme, the majority had a medical condition preventing them from doing so.

Health Outcomes

Outcome data from the CR programme have been collected routinely since the inception of the programme in Gloucestershire in 1992 (details of the questionnaires used to collect health-outcome data are given in Chapter 4). The most recently analysed data from 2006–7 (from the 778 patients who attended CR and completed questionnaires) showed the following outcomes:

- **Medication**—the NSF targets for the prescription of statins and Aspirin were met (NSF = 80–90 per cent of patients)

The health-outcome data showed significant improvement in the following areas:

- **Wellbeing**—Overall quality of life (>70 per cent improved)
- **Mental quality of life** (>61 per cent improved)
- **Physical quality of life** (>69 per cent improved)
- **Depression**—remained significantly reduced at one year post-cardiac event
- **Anxiety**—remained significantly reduced at one year post-cardiac event

At the end of CR:

- **Diet** — Significantly more people consumed three servings of fruit and vegetables a day (>62 per cent) and oily fish at least once a week (>86 per cent)
- **BMI** (body mass index)—78 per cent had a BMI of less than 30kg/m^2 (NSF = 75 per cent less than 30 kg/m^2)
- **Smoking**—87 per cent were not smoking, a continued improvement on previous years' figures (NSF = 75 per cent not smoking)
- **Exercise**—49 per cent reported exercising five times a week, for at least 30 minutes each time, continuing to improve upon the previous year's figures (and meeting the NSF target of 40 per cent of patients exercising five times week for 30 minutes)

Professional Development of the CR Team

The CR team in Gloucestershire has an integrated continuing professional development (CPD) programme ensuring that the service is delivered by appropriately trained and educated staff. Each member of the team takes part in an annual individual performance and development review (IPDR) and professional and service needs are identified through a personal development plan (PDP). CPD activities are then planned to meet individual needs and the needs of the service. Team members are supported in attending relevant training events, observational training opportunities and national conferences. Team members have undertaken service research and disseminated the findings at local, national and international conferences and in peer-reviewed journals, as well as guest lecturing at a variety of health professional teaching events across the UK.

Psychology and Cardiac Rehabilitation

Psychological Factors

In the remainder of this chapter we will look at some of the psychological factors (particularly illness perceptions) that are important following a cardiac event, and then describe how these factors influence the CR programme in Gloucestershire.

Experiencing a cardiac event and being diagnosed with coronary heart disease can come as a major shock for many patients, and it is therefore no surprise that the impact of the event and diagnosis can be far-reaching. Most patients will experience some degree of psychological distress following their cardiac event as a normal and understandable response to that event. For other patients, however, the event can challenge some of their previously held beliefs about their health (discussed below under "Illness perceptions") affecting how they respond both emotionally and behaviourally. The NSF for CR states that "after a major illness most people need some re-assurance and psychological support to help them regain their self-confidence" (Department of Health, 2000, ch. 7). Research into the psychological changes that occur after a major cardiac event such as a myocardial infarction or coronary artery bypass graft has shown that regaining self-confidence is only one of several psychological factors, such as anxiety (Lane et al., 2002; Mayou et al., 2000), depression (Frasure-Smith et al., 1993, 1995) and perceived control (Michie et al., 2005), that are of importance.

There has been little research into the psychological factors that might contribute to recovery and influence healthy behaviours following a cardiac event (Michie et al., 2005). Until recently, research into psychological factors following a cardiac event focused on affective states such as anxiety and depression (particularly after heart attack). Increasingly the role of illness perceptions and how patients make sense of their condition has become central in helping patients to understand and manage their rehabilitation more effectively.

Anxiety and Depression

Anxiety and depression are the most common psychological problems that occur following a cardiac event. Depression in particular has been found to be predictive of morbidity and mortality following a heart attack in major research studies. Frasure-Smith et al. (1993) found that major depression in patients in hospital after MI increased the risk of mortality for those patients in the first six months following their heart attack. Frasure-Smith also found that depression while in hospital following an MI was a significant predictor of 18-month post-MI cardiac mortality (Frasure-Smith et al., 1995). Mayou et al. (2000) studied anxiety and depression in 347 patients post-MI and found that those who were distressed in hospital were at high risk of adverse psychological and quality-of-life outcomes during the ensuing year. Studies focusing on CABG and psychological outcomes have also shown that psychological factors are important pre- and post-cardiac surgery. Herlitz et al. (1999) found that impaired physical and psychological quality of life before cardiac surgery predicted an impaired quality of life five years after CABG. Certain studies have shown depression to be common after cardiac surgery (Duits, 1996; Mayou, 1992), or that depression can worsen for some patients following CABG (Murphy et al., 2008). Other research has shown that psychological factors can have an important impact on recovery post-cardiac surgery. For instance, Stengrevics et al. (1996) found that pre-operative anxiety of patients waiting for cardiac surgery was predictive of post-operative outcome for these patients in terms of length of stay in hospital, number of complications post-surgery and clinical rating of surgical outcome.

Anxiety and depression are discussed in Week 6 of the CR group programme (within a cognitive behavioural model) and within the framework of "making the most of your recovery". Stress and coronary heart disease is discussed in Week 2 of the programme, and relaxation, as an element of stress (and/or anxiety) management, is also discussed in that week. Abdominal (or diaphragmatic) breathing for relaxation is taught in Week 2 of the programme, and a CD with three spoken relaxation techniques is given to patients and explained on Week 4 of the programme.

Psychological Factors and Health Outcomes

The research evidence suggests that psychological factors pre- and post-cardiac event are important in predicting health outcomes for cardiac patients. The impact of cardiac rehabilitation on these psychological factors and how this affects recovery after a cardiac event is less clear. As stated earlier, the NSF chapter for cardiac rehabilitation links psychological support after a cardiac event to regaining self-confidence. This is certainly an important aim of cardiac rehabilitation, yet the process of psychological change after a cardiac event, such as how and why patients regain confidence, is not clear. The impact of a cardiac event on an individual is both physical and psychological in nature, and because of this the cognitive, emotional, behavioural and physical changes that occur after a cardiac event, during CR and after CR interact in a complex way. Meta-analyses of exercise-only CR programmes for patients with coronary heart disease have shown a significant reduction in anxiety and depression for this client group (Kugler et al., 1994). This analysis showed that psychological change, measured by changes in anxiety and depression, is possible when patients engage in a physical exercise programme. Other studies (Milani et al., 1996) have shown similar results, and this has led to researchers becoming more interested in the processes of change after a cardiac event and following cardiac rehabilitation. In particular, the focus of much recent psychological research has been on patients' individual perceptions of their heart condition and how these so-called, "illness perceptions" may affect their physical and psychological recovery following a cardiac event.

Illness Perceptions

Research into how patients view their illness, or medical condition, has suggested that individuals categorise a particular condition through a set of themes or components known as "illness perceptions" (Leventhal et al., 1980). Leventhal and colleagues (Leventhal et al., 1980; Leventhal and Nerenz, 1985) proposed a self-regulatory model (SRM) of illness (or "common-sense model of illness") that seeks to explain how patients attempt to make sense of their condition and how this subsequently influences the way in which they cope with a particular condition. Leventhal suggests that when faced with an illness threat a patient will form illness perceptions, or representations, about their condition along the following five constructs:

- **Identity**—the label that an individual uses to describe their condition, e.g. "heart attack" or "coronary heart disease", and the symptoms that they associate with that condition
- **Cause**—personal ideas about the cause of the condition, e.g. smoking or stress
- **Timeline**—how long the individual believes that the illness will continue. "Is it an acute episode or a chronic condition?"
- **Consequences**—the expected consequences of the condition, physically, economically and socially
- **Cure/control**—how the individual believes he or she will recover from or control the condition

Leventhal et al. (1980) suggest, in the SRM, that patients use a framework of illness perceptions to make sense of their condition and in turn produce a coping response to manage their condition. Leventhal proposes that this processing system interacts with a parallel pathway involving an emotional response to the illness threat and a coping response to manage these emotions. Feedback loops allow the emotional response and the process of coping with this response to further influence coping with the original illness threat. Leventhal identified a number of coping strategies that are employed by patients:

- **Avoidance or denial**—e.g. "It was only a small MI so I don't need to attend cardiac rehabilitation . . ."
- **Cognitive reappraising**—e.g. "It's not so bad, with medical management and lifestyle change I'll be OK . . ."
- **Expressing emotions**—e.g. irritability, anger, crying, inappropriate humour
- **Problem-focused coping**—e.g. consulting with doctors, taking medicine, attending CR
- **Seeking social support**—e.g. talking with friends, family, CR professionals

These strategies will be reviewed and modified depending on how the patient views the progression of their illness. People with CHD can therefore develop a helpful framework of useful information and accurate illness perceptions that promotes confidence, healthy behaviours and adherence to treatment. Alternatively they may hold beliefs that are based on misconceptions that cause them, for example, to become fearful and adopt strategies that may appear inappropriate (such as not taking their medication or deciding not to attend CR).

The SRM has provided an attractive framework for researchers into a wide range of illnesses (Fortune et al., 2000; Moss-Morris, 1997; Murphy et al., 1999), and in particular the study of cardiac events where emotional responses such as anxiety and depression are common.

Illness Perceptions and Cardiac Events

Petrie et al. (1996) measured patients' illness perceptions when admitted to hospital with a first MI, and discovered that these illness perceptions predicted a number of outcomes. Petrie found that return to work within six weeks of the MI was significantly predicted by patients' illness perceptions that their condition would only last a short time (timeline) and would have less serious consequences for them (consequences). Furthermore, patients' beliefs that their heart condition would have serious consequences were significantly related to later disability in housework, recreational and social activities. A strong illness identity was related to greater sexual dysfunction at both three and six months post-MI. Petrie also found that patients' attendance at a CR programme was significantly related to a stronger belief during admittance that their condition could be controlled or cured (Petrie et al., 1996). Whitmarsh et al. (2003) investigated whether attendees at CR differed from non-attendees in relation to the illness perception framework of the SRM and whether any of the five components outlined by Leventhal in the SRM predicted attendance behaviours. This research reinforced the findings of Petrie et al. (1996), in that a weaker belief in the curability/controllability of the condition was the greatest predictor of poorer attendance or non-attendance at CR. Whitmarsh et al. also found differences between attendees and non-attendees, in that attendees perceived a greater number of symptoms and a greater number of consequences of their illness, suffered greater distress and held a wider range of beliefs about the cause of their condition (Whitmarsh et al., 2003).

Petrie et al. (2002) in a follow-up to the 1996 study which showed the importance of patients' illness perceptions in affecting their recovery, looked at whether an intervention designed to alter patients' perceptions of their MI would result in better recovery and reduced disability. The intervention involved 65 patients in hospital after their first MI who were randomly assigned to receive either three 30- to 40-minute assessment sessions with a psychologist aimed at altering incorrect or negative illness perceptions or standard in-hospital nurse visits and standard MI educational literature. Each individual in the intervention group received broadly the same intervention, although the exact content was finalised using results from their scores on the Illness Perception Questionnaire (IPQ) (Weinman et al., 1996). This questionnaire was developed to provide a quantitative measure of illness perceptions, and in particular the five components of the SRM: identity, cause, consequences, timeline and control/cure. In the first assessment session the psychologist outlined the patho-physiology of an MI using drawings, explained terminology and described common symptoms of MI, making a distinction between cardiac and non-cardiac symptoms. This session also explored the patient's beliefs about the cause of their MI and in particular it aimed to broaden the patient's beliefs around the involvement of lifestyle factors in the aetiology of their CHD and their subsequent MI. The second assessment session built on the causal factors identified in session one and aimed to develop a plan to minimise future risk by reducing risk factors and increasing control over the condition (Petrie et al., 2002). Using scores obtained from the timeline and consequences subscales of the IPQ, a written action plan was developed to include exercise, dietary change and return to work (if appropriate), once negative beliefs about long-term consequences of the MI had been challenged. In the third assessment session the action plan was reviewed and symptoms of recovery were discussed, as were concerns about medication and returning home (Petrie et al., 2002). Patients were followed up at three months post-discharge, where information was collected regarding returning to work, symptoms of angina and illness perceptions. Illness perceptions were measured using the IPQ when patients enrolled on the study, then again at discharge from hospital and once again at three-month follow-up. Petrie et al. found that the intervention led to significant positive changes in patients' illness perceptions about their MI. They found that patients in the intervention group, on leaving hospital, had modified, positive perceptions of how long their condition would last (timeline) and how serious the consequences of their condition would be for them. The intervention group also showed a stronger belief that their illness could be controlled or cured. The changes in timeline and control/cure were maintained at the three-month follow-up. Petrie et al. also found that patients in the intervention group reported that they were better prepared to leave hospital and that they returned to work sooner than patients in the control group. At three-month follow-up the patients from the intervention group reported a significantly lower rate of angina symptoms than patients from the usual-care group, showing that an intervention designed to change patients' illness perceptions could also result in improved functional outcome following an MI (Petrie et al., 2002).

The studies of Petrie et al. (1996, 2002) have shown that patients' illness perceptions can positively influence their recovery, both in relation to behaviours, such as returning to work, and to their physical recovery following a heart attack. The intervention study (Petrie et al., 2002) showed that patients' illness perceptions can change over time, and that these changes can positively affect their physical recovery, as measured by a reduction in angina symptoms following MI. This has implications for cardiac rehabilitation programmes, as the aim of CR as outlined in the NSF is to help patients to "achieve the lifestyle changes they want to make", and to, "enjoy the best possible physical, mental and emotional health and so return to as full and normal a life as possible" (Department of Health, 2000). By understanding the mechanisms that enable patients to engage in positive health behaviours following a cardiac event, CR programmes are better able to target interventions to patients.

Illness Perceptions and CR

At present there has been little research looking at the effect of cardiac rehabilitation itself on patients' illness perceptions and how these may change pre- and post-cardiac rehabilitation. Michie et al. (2005) studied the mechanisms of psychological change that occur following CR, and how these changes may impact on recovery. Sixty-two patients were followed up eight weeks after the end of their comprehensive CR programme, and 29 of these patients were followed up again at eight months post-CR. Patients completed the IPQ before attending the CR programme, and then again before attending both of the follow-ups. They also completed the Hospital Anxiety and Depression Scale (Zigmond and Snaith, 1983) and the SF-12 (Ware et al., 1996), a 12-item quality-of-life scale that measures physical and mental functioning, at all three of these time points. At eight weeks and at eight months post-CR patients showed increased perceived control over their condition, decreased anxiety and depression, and more confidence in changing their eating habits (Michie et al., 2005). The increase in perceived control predicted anxiety and depression at eight-week follow-up. The decrease in depression predicted lower anxiety at eight weeks and lower anxiety and depression and better mental health at eight months. Lowered anxiety predicted lower depression at eight weeks but also lowered anxiety and depression and a trend towards better physical health at eight months (Michie et al., 2005). The conclusion from this research is that the increased sense of perceived control over their condition that patients report following CR may impact on levels of distress (anxiety and depression), which may in turn have long-term benefits for both physical and mental health. The relatively small sample size and the absence of a control group means that the findings cannot be attributed directly to the CR programme. However, the authors state that the changes taking place appear to be "due to changes in illness perceptions, in particular perceptions of control and emotional changes rather than any alternative mechanism" (Michie et al., 2005).

The importance of illness perceptions in affecting recovery after MI (Petrie et al., 1996, 2002), recovery after cardiac rehabilitation (Michie et al., 2005) and influencing attendance at cardiac rehabilitation (Whitmarsh et al., 2003) has been shown in recent research. Different illness perceptions have been implicated in influencing different health behaviours and in influencing aspects of physical and mental recovery (Michie et al., 2005; Petrie et al., 1996, 2002; Whitmarsh et al., 2003). However, it has been proposed that perceived control over the condition may be the most important illness perception following CR (Michie et al., 2005). *Perceived* control is one of several psychological theories of control that has been proposed.

Control Theory

Control theory has become an important concept in the psychology of health, and has important applications in the fields of chronic health and rehabilitation. Perceived control refers to the extent to which a situation is believed to be "under control" (Walker, 2001). Walker uses the example of how a situation may be perceived to be "under control" without any direct influence from the individual, such as when responsibility for an event is shared within a team. This example can be directly related to post-MI care in hospital, where a patient may believe, for example, that "the medical team" has their health-care situation "under control". By contrast, personal control is based on the individual's direct influence over an event. A further definition: perceived personal control refers to the individual's *belief* that things are under their direct control. The concepts of perceived control, personal control and perceived personal control have been seen as increasingly important within health-care settings, and have been shown to influence and predict a number of health outcomes (Michie et al., 2005; Turk et al., 1995; Wallston et al., 1987). It is the concept of perceived control (over a specific health condition) that has been suggested by Michie et al. (2005) to be the theoretical control construct that has the most direct relevance to recovery following CR. The suggestion is that the increased sense of perceived control over their cardiac condition that patients experience following CR has an impact on levels of distress (anxiety and depression) which subsequently has a positive impact on physical and emotional recovery.

Applying Psychological Theory in CR

The research tells us that there are a number of psychological factors that are important to patients following a cardiac event (anxiety, stress, depression, perceived control) and that are therefore of importance in the development and implementation of CR programmes. The psychological input to the CR programme in Gloucestershire begins long before patients arrive for their first session of the group programme.

Anxiety at Assessment

Anxiety is the earliest and most common response to a cardiac event. As MI patients are assessed (assessments are described in more detail in Chapter 3) on the cardiac wards in Gloucestershire within a few days of their cardiac event, it is no surprise that many are found to have high levels of anxiety. As anxiety is a normal response to a potentially life-threatening event, this anxiety is acknowledged at assessment but does not form the rationale for intervention. A patient who is extremely distressed may be referred to the cardiac psychologist for further assessment, but otherwise a degree of anxiety would be expected. Some patients may become euphoric on realising that they have survived a heart attack, but this is often replaced by the realisation that their condition may have negative implications for their life and their future. As people deal with emotions differently some patients may present as distressed, tearful or frightened, whereas others may repeatedly ask questions without appearing to retain information (anxiety can affect memory, concentration and attention), or deny or question their diagnosis. As high levels of anxiety will often be driven by misconceptions or unhelpful beliefs about their condition, of major potential interest to the assessor will be the patients' illness perceptions, especially those concerning "cause" and "timeline". These beliefs about the cause of the patient's condition are important, as they are established in the first few weeks following a cardiac event and become increasingly resistant to change.

Illness Perceptions at Assessment

The assessment is a golden opportunity to broaden patients' thinking about what has caused their cardiac event and to begin to link their understanding of their event to the concept of coronary heart disease as a chronic condition. In Gloucestershire, a 45-minute assessment may start with questions relating to an individual's understanding of what caused their condition and then move through a description of CHD, its symptoms and management, followed by a detailed assessment of the individual's CHD risk factors (see Chapter 3). Initial misconceptions can then be carefully challenged. As many patients will only remember a fraction of the information given at assessment, a booklet with information relating to CHD, its risk factors and its management is given to the patient to read and take home. This information should be consistent with information given at assessment. Misconceptions can arise from ambiguous messages given by health professionals as well as from lay sources (e.g. "If you take it easy you should be fine" may be interpreted as, "activity is dangerous for me and should therefore be avoided"). It is important to check that patients understand the information that has been given to them to ensure that misconceptions have not arisen at the assessment.

Returning Home

When a patient returns home following their cardiac event it is often the time when the full implications of their event become clear. The effect of the cardiac event and a period of inactivity in hospital (causing deconditioning) will often leave patients feeling weaker than they expected. As a result patients may have active and shifting beliefs about the short- and long-term consequences of their condition ("Will I ever return to normal?" or "Will I have another MI and die?"). In an attempt to make sense of, and adjust to, their condition, patients can be vulnerable to misconceptions. These misconceptions, often about the cause and prognosis of their condition, can hinder recovery and are closely related to increased levels of psychological distress. It is therefore essential that the information provided to patients when leaving hospital is clear, accurate and consistently reinforced throughout their patient journey to avoid developing or reinforcing harmful misconceptions.

The CR Group

The Gloucestershire group CR programme uses a cognitive behavioural framework, emphasising the links between thoughts, emotions, physical responses and behaviours. This is particularly to the fore in Week 1 ("Impact of a Cardiac

Event"), Week 2 ("Stress") and Week 6 ("Making the Most of Your Recovery"). For a good introduction to the cognitive behavioural approach see White (2001).

The programme is also underpinned by a number of health psychology models, including self-regulatory theory (discussed earlier in this chapter), Lazarus' transactional model of stress, the transtheoretical model, and the theory of planned behaviour (for a good introduction to these models see Ogden, 2007). The goal-setting and pacing approach that is presented in Week 1 of the programme was initially developed for the management of individuals with chronic pain

Self-regulatory theory and illness perception remain important when a patient attends the CR group programme in Gloucestershire, as increasing patients' perceived control through CR appears to be one of the most important factors in affecting recovery following a cardiac event (Michie et al., 2005).

Attending a CR group programme allows patients to educate themselves about CHD and its management and to learn how to exercise at a level that is correct for them following their cardiac event (the practical aspects of this will be considered in detail in Chapters 5 to 11). However, the exercise programme and the provision of accurate information (both about exercise and about the medical aspects) on the CR programme can also have an impact on patients' illness perceptions. Some patients arrive at Week 1 of the CR programme with a good understanding of coronary heart disease, its risk factors and the chronic nature of their condition. Others may still hold misconceptions about their condition that can have a profound effect on their illness perceptions and their recovery. Week 1 of the CR programme aims to challenge some of the potential misconceptions that patients may have by discussing CHD in detail and describing how it can be managed by medical intervention and medication and through lifestyle factors. A common cure/control misconception for patients arriving at CR is that having left hospital (perhaps following an intervention such as angioplasty or CABG) they are "cured". These patients may then believe that there is little or no point in taking their medication, or that there is little point coming to CR. This type of misconception can be gently challenged in the first week of the programme. Misconceptions are challenged throughout the group programme, both individually with patients and through talks that are given about medication, stress, angina, blood pressure and diet and CHD.

As mentioned previously in this chapter, it appears that patients' sense of perceived control over their condition is enhanced following CR, and that this improved sense of control impacts positively on their recovery. This is evident in the area of exercise, where it is often the case that engaging in the exercise programme challenges patients' illness perceptions. Many have not exercised for lengthy periods of time and may believe that exercise needs to be strenuous to be of any benefit. Many patients are apprehensive about exercising (for the first time in months or even years for some patients), and may be worried about exercising in a group environment. Some patients may believe themselves to be fitter than they are and may push themselves beyond their limits to demonstrate this. Other patients inevitably compare themselves to the person exercising next to them. These comparisons can lead to increased confidence ("I'm not as bad as them") but may also shock patients into realising that they are actually worse than they thought. However it appears that for many patients their control beliefs are increased through the medium of exercising in a paced way on CR and in a safe environment (this is described in more detail in Chapter 3).

Chapter 3
The Exercise Programme

This chapter describes the exercise programme that is an integral part of the multidisciplinary cardiac rehabilitation programme in Gloucestershire. We have included details of the exercise programme in this chapter rather than in the subsequent chapters that describe the CR programme both to avoid repetition and for ease of reference for those wishing to consider this aspect of CR in isolation.

Risk Stratification for Exercise

One of the standard interventions for patients in CR is the prescription of a structured exercise programme, while encouraging individuals to increase their daily physical activity levels (Williams, 2001). There is strong evidence to support the use of formal exercise training in the management and secondary prevention of coronary heart disease (Taylor et al., 2004). The reported incidence of adverse events during CR exercise training is low. In a 16-year follow-up, Franklin et al. (1998) reported that the incidence of major cardiovascular events during exercise ranged from 1 in 50,000 to 1 in 120,000 patient hours of exercise and two fatalities in 1.5 million patient hours of exercise. More recent data suggest similar outcomes, with a risk of non-fatal events in 1 in 58,000 hours of exercise per year (Scheinowitz and Harpaz, 2005).

Before commencing a cardiac rehabilitation programme, all patients need to be risk-stratified. Risk stratification is the process of estimating the risk that an individual has of developing acute cardiovascular complications during an exercise session. The criteria are derived from research that considers factors that are associated with increased mortality and morbidity.

Risk-stratification decisions in CR in Gloucestershire are based on a number of clinical criteria taken from the American Association of Cardiovascular and Pulmonary Rehabilitation (AACVPR) and are outlined below:

1. **Characteristics of patients at the lowest risk for exercise participation (all characteristics listed must be present for the patient to remain at the lowest risk)**
   - Absence of complex ventricular arrhythmias during exercise testing and recovery

- Absence of angina or other significant symptoms (e.g. unusual shortness of breath, light-headedness, or dizziness during exercise testing and recovery)
- Presence of normal hemodynamics during exercise testing and recovery (i.e. an appropriate increase and subsequent decrease in heart rate and systolic blood pressure with increasing workload and recovery)
- Functional capacity $\geq$ 7 METS. METS, or Metabolic equivalents, are a simplified system for classifying physical activities where one MET is equal to the resting oxygen consumption, which is approximately 3.5 millilitres of oxygen per kilogram of body weight (3.5 ml/kg/min)

Non-exercise testing findings:

- Rest ejection fraction $\geq$ 50 per cent
- Uncomplicated MI or revasculisation procedure
- Absence of complicated ventricular arrhythmias at rest
- Absence of congestive heart failure
- Absence of signs and symptoms of post-event/post-procedure ischaemia
- Absence of clinical depression

2. **Characteristics of patients at moderate risk for exercise participation (any one or combination of these findings places a person at moderate risk; see Table 3.1)**

- Presence of angina or other significant symptoms (e.g. unusual shortness of breath, light-headedness, or dizziness occurring at high levels of exertion [$\geq$ 7 METS])
- Mild to moderate level of silent ischaemia during exercise testing or recovery (ST-segment depression < 2 mm from baseline)
- Functional capacity < 5 METS)

Non-exercise test findings:

- Rest ejection fraction = 40–49 per cent

3. **Characteristics of patients at high risk for exercise participation (any one or combination of these findings places a person at high risk)**

- Presence of complex ventricular arrhythmias during exercise testing and recovery
- Presence of angina or other significant symptoms (e.g. unusual shortness of breath, light-headedness, or dizziness occurring at low levels of exertion [< 5 METS] or during recovery)
- High level of silent ischaemia recovery (ST-segment depression $\geq$ 2 mm from baseline) during exercise testing or recovery
- Presence of abnormal hemodynamics during exercise testing (i.e. chronotrophic incompetence or flat or decreasing systolic blood pressure with increasing workloads) or recovery (i.e. severe post-exercise hypotension)

Non-exercise test findings:

- Resting ejection fraction < 40 per cent
- History of cardiac arrest, or sudden death

- Complex dysrhythmias at rest
- Complicated MI or revascularisation procedure
- Presence of chronic heart failure (CHF)
- Presence or signs and symptoms of post-event/post-procedure ischaemia
- Presence of clinical depression

AACVPR Stratification of Risk for Cardiac Events during Exercise
Participation (Williams and Balady, 1999)

The details above describe the criteria used for the risk stratification on the CR programme. Having just one factor in the high-risk category would put that individual at a high risk even if all the other factors were low-risk.

It is important to note that a change in a patient's condition during the CR programme may require an alteration to their risk-stratification level. This is especially common in situations where patients are having ongoing investigations or treatments while attending the CR programme.

Using the Information

Once a risk-stratification decision has been made, we need to decide how the information will be used. There are a number of ways in which this risk-stratification information could potentially be used:

- High-risk patients may need to be treated at a higher ratio to low-risk patients, i.e. 1:5 for low-risk and 1:3 for high-risk.
- In some instances it is not possible to accept high-risk patients onto community-based CR programmes, and they can only attend hospital-based rehabilitation. This will depend on the type of resuscitation support available at each venue. For example, if you have a community venue with good ambulance response times or resuscitation equipment on site it may be deemed appropriate to accept high-risk patients onto the group. However,

Table 3.1 Example of a moderate-risk patient

50-year-old patient

Recent history of inferior myocardial infarction and subsequent angioplasty to right coronary artery

Echocardiogram result—moderate left ventricular (LV) function with estimated ejection fraction (EF) 47%

No current angina or ischaemia

No exercise test result

No arrhythmias

No presence of heart failure

This patient would be classed as a ***moderate risk*** due to their moderate LV function and EF of 47%

a high-risk patient may be more suitable for a hospital-run CR programme in areas where ambulance response times are slow (such as rural locations) or resuscitation equipment is not available.

- High-risk patients can be advised to work at a lower intensity (such as keeping their heart rate at 50–60 per cent of its maximum rather than the 60–75 per cent currently used in Phase III rehabilitation).

Supervision Following Exercise

The Association of Chartered Physiotherapists in Cardiac Rehabilitation (ACPICR) and the BACR suggest that patients should be supervised for between 15 and 30 minutes following cessation of exercise. This is to monitor for post-exercise complications such as hypotension or arrhythmias. Exercise should therefore ideally occur at the start of the CR session and any educational aspects should follow the exercise session.

Exercise Practical Sessions

There is no substitute for getting practical exercise experience under the supervision of trained health professionals. Having a cardiac event can be a frightening experience for both patients and their immediate family. Patients may need a great deal of support to get back to their normal exercise routine and to return to work and other physical activities. The exercise practical component of cardiac rehabilitation should complement the educational information given on the programme.

It should be noted that we use a form of interval (rather than intermittent) exercise in CR classes. A large percentage of patients who come along to CR programmes can be severely deconditioned and are not able to manage continuous periods of cardiovascular exercise for lengthy periods of time.

Typically on a CR programme there can be a wide age range of patients, and thus the exercise component needs to cater for a wide range of abilities and fitness levels. The use of circuit-based exercise programmes is common in CR because it can give the freedom to manage a mixed-ability group while catering for large patient numbers. The typical staff-to-patient ratio is 1:5 for low-risk clients; however, if there is a greater number of high-risk clients this may increase to 1:3.

Calculating Heart-Rate Training Ranges

Before commencing a practical exercise session patients should have an individual heart-rate training range calculated for them. There are two main

Table 3.2 Maximum heart rate

220-age (further 20–30 beats if on beta-blockers) = maximum heart rate
60–75% of maximum heart rate is calculated to form a training range
e.g. A 55-year-old patient on beta-blockers would be calculated as follows:
   $220 - 55(-20) = 145$ bpm
   $0.60 \times 145 = 87$ bpm
   $0.75 \times 145 = 109$ bpm   **Training range = 87–109 bpm**

methods for calculating a training heart rate (see Tables 3.2 and 3.3). The discrepancy between the two readings shown in the tables is because the heart rate reserve method also takes into account the resting heart rate of the patient.

The maximum heart rate of an individual can be 10 beats above or below the estimated value using 220-age. Both methods are just an estimation of heart-rate training and should be used in conjunction with the Perceived Rate of Exercise Scale (see below).

It should be noted that patients who are severely deconditioned may be unable to maintain this level of exertion and may need to start at a lower training range and build up gradually over the duration of the programme.

Exercise Practical

Exercise Set-up

Before commencing a practical exercise session a full risk-stratification assessment should be completed for each patient to establish their individual risk of a further cardiac event during exercise.

Table 3.3 Heart rate reserve

220-age (further 20–30 beats if on beta-blockers) = maximum heart rate (MHR)
MHR − resting heart rate (RHR) = heart rate reserve (HRR)
$0.4 \times$ HRR + RHR = lower training range
$0.7 \times$ HRR + RHR = upper training range
e.g. A 55-year-old patient with a resting heart rate of 60 bpm would be calculated as follows:
   $220 - 55(-20) = 145$ bpm
   $145 - 60 = 85$ bpm (HRR)
   $0.4 \times 85 + 60 = 94$
   $0.7 \times 85 + 60 = 119$ **Training range = 94–119 bpm**

At the beginning of each exercise session it is advisable to check the following:

- Has the patient had any symptoms (e.g. angina) in the last week?
- Has their medication changed?
- Are they feeling well today?
- Have they brought their GTN (glyceryl trinitrate) to the session with them?

The following are *absolute* contraindications to exercise in Phase III CR:

- Fever or systemic illness
- Symptomatic hypotension
- Resting systolic blood pressure >200 mmHg or resting diastolic blood pressure >110 mmHg
- Resting heart rate above 100 bpm
- Acute or unstable heart failure
- Uncontrolled diabetes
- Uncontrolled or new arrhythmias
- Unstable angina

Warm-up

A group warm-up lasting at least 15 minutes should be completed before progressing to the main exercise component of the session. This should allow adequate time for patients' coronary arteries to dilate, and reduce the possibility of a patient experiencing an angina attack.

The warm-up should include:

- Joint mobility exercises
- Pulse-raising activities
- Upper and lower limb stretches

The warm-up should be simple and easy to follow. A chair or bar may be used for balance if this is an issue for a patient.

Circuit Exercise

Utilising a circuit programme as the main component of the exercise session allows for easy management of a mixed-ability group. There are a number of different formats that can be used depending on the space and equipment available at a venue.

Interval training involves alternating between cardiovascular and active recovery exercises. One of the main advantages of active recovery work is that it allows a longer total duration of exercise and allows easier management of a mixed-ability group.

Cardiovascular (CV) Exercise	Exercise involving large rhythmical movements of the arms and the legs
Active Recovery (AR)	Either an exercise that involves lower-intensity work than the cardiovascular exercise or an alternative activity that allows some recovery

It is also important not to encourage complete rest during an exercise session as patients can be at risk of postural hypotension. Sudden changes in heart rate and blood pressure can leave patients at risk of arrhythmias.

The examples below show how circuit programmes can be designed to manage differing exercise abilities.

Figure 3.1 shows the CV exercises located around the edge of the room and the AR exercises located in the centre of the room. Patients would be given a level to work at which would guide how often they go into the centre of the room to the AR station.

This type of circuit design should only be used if there is enough equipment available to allow a number of people to be at the stations simultaneously. The circuit can be managed by a whistle, or by a break in the exercise music

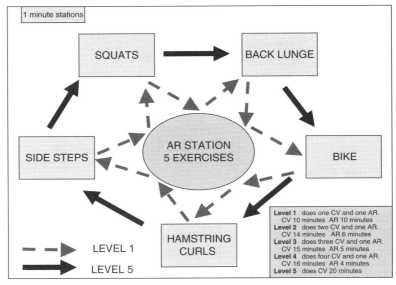

Figure 3.1 Cardiovascular and active recovery exercises

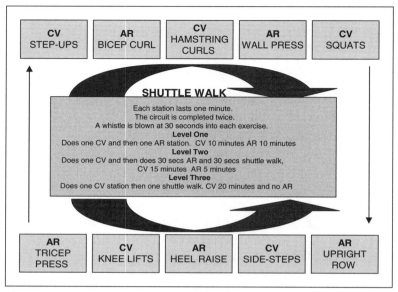

| CV STEP-UPS | AR BICEP CURL | CV HAMSTRING CURLS | AR WALL PRESS | CV SQUATS |

SHUTTLE WALK

Each station lasts one minute.
The circuit is completed twice.
A whistle is blown at 30 seconds into each exercise.
Level One
Does one CV and then one AR station. CV 10 minutes AR 10 minutes
Level Two
Does one CV and then does 30 secs AR and 30 secs shuttle walk,
CV 15 minutes AR 5 minutes
Level Three
Does one CV station then one shuttle walk. CV 20 minutes and no AR

| AR TRICEP PRESS | CV KNEE LIFTS | AR HEEL RAISE | CV SIDE-STEPS | AR UPRIGHT ROW |

Figure 3.2 Fast shuttle walk

occurring every minute. All of the patients will move around the circuit at the same time but can be going to different exercise stations.

Figure 3.2 utilises a fast shuttle walk as a cardiovascular exercise. Patients move around the circuit in a clockwise direction. At a basic level they would alternate between CV and AR exercises. As they progress they gradually replace AR with a shuttle walk, with the ultimate aim of doing all CV exercise.

Figure 3.3 shows how AR exercises (light grey boxes) can be altered to make them CV by adding larger arm and leg movements (dark grey boxes). For example Exercise 2 only involves raising heels and pushing arms behind the body, which is a recovery exercise. By adding a step backwards this becomes a CV exercise.

The ultimate aim with all of the circuit designs is to allow a gradual progression from interval training to continuous cardiovascular exercise.

Tips for Class Management

• Keep the duration of each exercise the same to avoid confusion when moving around the exercises
• Set out the exercises so that the patients are clearly visible
• If possible have more than one piece of equipment available at each station
• Check heart rates on a CV exercise rather than on an AR exercise (where it may be lower)

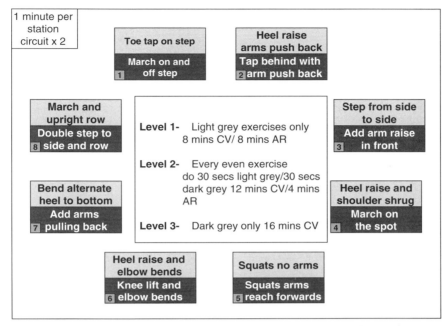

Figure 3.3 Altering active recovery exercises to make them cardiovascular

Muscle Balance

When designing an exercise circuit the "muscle balance" of the circuit should be considered. Typically, circuit programmes overuse the quadricep muscles at the expense of other muscle groups. Consider having exercises that work other muscles groups, such as the hip abductors/adductors and hamstrings.

The exercises on the left-hand side of Figure 3.4 show how a series of them can over-emphasise the quadricep muscles. The exercises on the right contain a better balance by including alternative muscle groups.

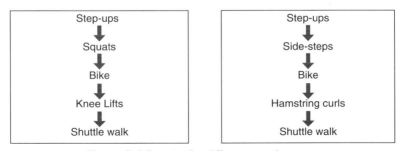

Figure 3.4 Exercise for different muscle groups

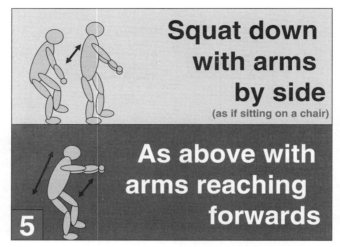

Figure 3.5 Card for use in an exercise circuit

Exercise Cards

Having clearly printed exercise cards that are simple and easy to read will help in teaching the exercises to the patients. Ideally the exercise cards will consist of a diagram of a particular exercise with simple text written above or below, explaining the exercise. This should help patients' understanding of the exercises (the text should be of an adequate size to read from a distance). Figure 3.5 shows an example of an exercise card that has been developed for use in an exercise circuit.

Cool-down

A group cool-down should last at least 10 minutes to allow adequate time for a patient's heart rate and blood pressure to return to normal. In an older patient population the baroreceptors (pressure sensors) become less receptive and thus it takes the body longer to make changes to blood pressure.

Having an adequate cool-down is also important in reducing the risk of post-exercise hypotension or arrhythmias.

The format of the cool-down should be similar to the warm-up, but in reverse, to include pulse-lowering activities, mobility work and muscle stretches.

Use of Music

The decision regarding the use of music tends to be a personal one!

Advantages of Exercising to Music

- Enjoyable (for some!)
- Keep to a continuous beat
- Can be split up to aid timing at each station (e.g. a gap in the music after one minute)

Disadvantages of Exercising to Music

- Can be too fast for people to keep up with
- Difficult to hear exercise instructions
- Different tastes in music

If you choose to use music during a practical exercise session make sure that the volume is kept to a suitable level so that your voice can be heard easily, and that the choice of music is appropriate to the age range of the patient group!

Gym Programmes

Depending on the location of the programme you may have access to gym equipment. Gym equipment can be utilised as a group gym programme (the same as the circuit but using the gym equipment) or by setting each patient an individual gym programme. There are relative merits to both of these options. Individual programmes will allow a specific prescription for that client but does not allow for group interaction. Group programmes may be more difficult for the exercise professional to manage but will allow a greater degree of bonding between individual patients.

Seated Exercises

Some patients may be unable to manage standing exercises due to other health conditions. Rather than excluding these patients from exercise completely, an alternative exercise circuit, that can be completed from a chair (or using a chair or bar for support), may be offered. The relative intensity of this exercise is likely to be considerably lower in terms of heart rate but some individuals can gain great benefit for their general mobility (as well as the other positive benefits that come from participating in a group session).

Chapter 4
Preparing for the First Session

This chapter will describe some of the practicalities of setting up and running a CR programme. This will include details of the multidisciplinary team (MDT), staff training, recruitment, referral, assessment, patient invitation to the CR programme and the questionnaires used to collect health-outcome data. Details of the suitability of venues and the equipment needed to deliver CR will also be discussed.

The multidisciplinary cardiac rehabilitation team in Gloucestershire consists of cardiac nurses, clinical and health psychologists, physiotherapists, exercise specialists and dieticians. Each group programme is delivered by a nurse, exercise professional or physiotherapist and psychologist, with all three attending each session. Attention is given to the skill mix within the team so that wherever possible junior members are teamed up with senior members at each venue. The most senior member has the responsibility for managing the programme at that venue and taking any immediate decisions relating to health and safety, staff or patient issues.

Staff Background and Training

All of the nurses working in cardiac rehabilitation in Gloucestershire are registered with the Nursing and Midwifery Council with a willingness to undertake an appropriate teaching/assessing qualification. They also have a minimum of two years' experience of cardiology nursing.

Psychologists are either chartered health or clinical psychologists, or are trainee psychologists under supervision. All members of the team are trained in Cognitive Behavioural Therapy.

Physiotherapists have a BSc Honours degree in physiotherapy and ideally have a qualification through the Association of Chartered Physiotherapists in Cardiac Rehabilitation (ACPICR). The exercise professionals are British Association for Cardiac Rehabilitation (BACR) Phase IV-trained.

All staff are routinely trained and updated in resuscitation/life support.

In addition to the professional training relevant to their own discipline, inter-team training is provided via countywide CR team meetings, which are held twice yearly. In order to ensure effective multidisciplinary working, each discipline within the team has offered training to the other professionals within the MDT. For example, nurses have offered teaching on the medical aspects of coronary heart disease, the interventions for CHD and a session on heart failure. The psychologists have taught on the psychological models that underpin the CR programme, motivational interviewing, research carried out using patient data from the CR group programme and patient-centred assessments. The exercise team has taught on various aspects of exercise delivered on the CR programme.

When a new member of the team is recruited, a standard induction process is followed. This includes shadowing other CR professionals, both within their own discipline and the other disciplines within the MDT. They also observe two complete CR group programmes (with different staff teams delivering the programmes and preferably at different venues), attend team meetings with colleagues within their discipline and undergo individual supervision with a senior member of their team.

As feedback is an important part of effective multidisciplinary working, team members will routinely feed back to each other at the end of each week of the group programme. Feedback includes comments on individual talks or the management of group dynamics. When teams are well established, this becomes informal verbal feedback. However, when a new member joins a team at a venue, formal feedback forms are completed by all team members. Comments are offered on what went well and what could be improved within a session. Good communication ensures the smooth running of the team.

Team members are also trained in inpatient and outpatient assessment. Time is spent observing other team members assessing patients, and team members are then observed themselves. Although the assessment process is as standardised as possible, it is useful for any member of staff to observe how the various disciplines within the team assess patients differently (for example, to see how a psychologist deals with an anxious or distressed patient, or how a physiotherapist responds to exercise-related questions).

Eligibility for CR Group Programmes

Patients can be referred to the group CR programme in Gloucestershire either post-acute admission with an MI, following a diagnosis of angina or acute coronary syndrome, following an angioplasty, or having undergone a CABG. Patients who are excluded from group CR are typically too frail to attend, have significant problems with their cardiac health, have other co-morbidity, or are unable to travel to the community venues (e.g. individuals who are housebound in nursing homes or sheltered accommodation).

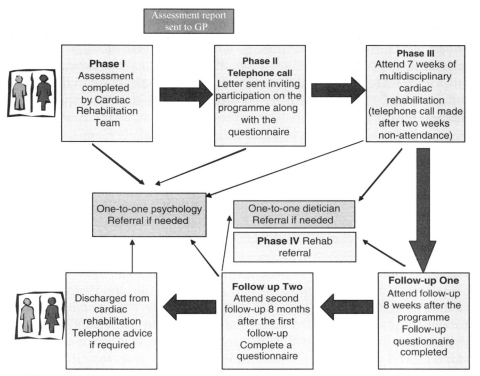

Figure 4.1 Flow diagram to illustrate a patient's journey through cardiac rehabilitation

The Patient Pathway

The CR patient journey is outlined in Figure 4.1.

Assessment

Inpatient Assessment

Following an acute admission, the CR team waits for the patient's condition to stabilise and for their diagnosis to be confirmed. It is the preference of the team not to assess patients in the Coronary Care Unit, wherever possible, as patient anxiety levels can be high and information given to the patient is often not retained. Patients are given the information booklet, "Understanding your Coronary Heart Disease", which includes explanations of coronary heart disease and its interventions, information on risk factors and lifestyle change, how to pace activities, current driving regulations and dietary information. The CR team member will then carry out a standardised assessment (see Appendix 1 for an example of an assessment document). Typically, this will begin by offering the patient the opportunity to tell their story, to explain the circumstances that have led up to their admission and for the assessor to ascertain the perceived cause of their CHD. The CHD process is then explained, along with a detailed explanation of the particular cardiac event that the patient has experienced. Risk factors relevant to the individual are identified, and the assessor will begin linking these risk factors to the disease process. At this stage the main aim is to give clear information to the patient in order to correct any misconceptions that they may hold about coronary heart disease or its management.

As the assessment progresses, information regarding national targets for blood pressure and cholesterol is given and guidance on pacing activities and exercise is offered. Explanations of cardiac medications are given, dietary advice is offered and onward referral to the smoking cessation service is made if and when appropriate. Instruction is given on monitoring and responding to chest pain alongside the use of the GTN protocol.

Finally the CR assessor will discuss the CR group programme, explaining its function, and will offer the patient the opportunity to attend the programme (if it is appropriate for them to do so). This can be an important opportunity to correct any misconceptions that the patient may have about CR groups, for example that cardiac rehabilitation is "just about exercise", or that it is a "support" group. Once the patient has chosen the venue most suitable for them and has agreed to attend, they are informed that the CR team will contact them in due course by letter inviting them to attend a group. Each patient is also offered a Phase II telephone call (preferably to be made within three working days of discharge from hospital) by a CR team member who will check that they are well and coping at home.

Patient Invitation

The patient invitation letter (see Appendix 2) is based on research that was carried out by the Gloucestershire CR team in 2001. In a randomised controlled trial it was shown that an invitation letter based on the theory of planned behaviour could increase attendance at cardiac rehabilitation programmes (Wyer et al., 2001). The letter has been adapted and used since 2001.

Measurement of Outcomes

Audit and evaluation should be a routine part of any good practice. In Gloucestershire the CR team have measured a variety of CR outcomes since 1992, enabling the service to monitor the efficacy of the CR group programme. The service is currently working towards submitting data to the National Audit for Cardiac Rehabilitation (NACR). Evaluation questionnaires are routinely given to patients at three time points:

1. Pre-programme questionnaire

Patients are sent a first questionnaire with their invitation letter and asked to complete it and bring it to the first week of the CR programme. At this time point, patients are assessed using a combination of standardised assessment questionnaires and theoretically informed questions. The current baseline measures are:

- The Hospital Anxiety and Depression Scale (Zigmond and Snaith, 1983)
- The Brief Illness Perception Questionnaire (Broadbent et al., 2006)
- The SF-12—Quality of Life Measure (Jenkinson and Layte, 1997)

There are also questions regarding:

- Medication
- Height and weight
- Smoking
- Physical exercise: frequency and intensity
- Work and employment
- Lifestyle change
- Eating and drinking

2. First follow-up questionnaire (eight weeks post-group completion)

Patients are sent a second questionnaire along with their invitation letter to attend a follow-up session, eight weeks after completing the CR programme. They are invited to complete the questionnaire at home, prior to attending the follow-up, and to bring the questionnaire with them to the follow-up session. All of the measures and questions listed above in the "Pre-programme questionnaire" are assessed again, in order to measure change over time. In addition, patients are invited to comment on various aspects of the programme, including the convenience of the location, the timing of the sessions, the content of the course and the quality of staff facilitation. Space is also provided for qualitative feedback about how to improve the programme.

3. Second follow-up questionnaire (approximately six months post-first follow up)

The second follow-up questionnaire is sent with an invitation to a second follow-up session, approximately six months after the first follow-up. This session will be approximately 12 months after the patients' cardiac event and allows for data collection at 12 months post-event in line with the NSF requirements. This questionnaire is the same as the first follow-up questionnaire minus the detailed feedback on the various aspects of the programme. Patients are invited to comment on what went well during their CR programme, what did not go so well and what could be improved.

Timing of CR

Typically, patients will be invited to attend a CR group no earlier than four weeks post-MI and CABG (in accordance with NSF guidelines). As there is a rolling timetable of group programmes in Gloucestershire, patients select their preferred venue and are allocated a CR place at that venue as soon as one becomes available. In order to make the groups as accessible as possible to patients, morning and afternoon groups are run at a range of venues across the county.

Open/Closed Groups

There are various models of group CR. Some CR services run open groups continuously and patients can opt in or out of the group as they choose. These are particularly well suited to stand-alone exercise rehabilitation programmes. As the Gloucestershire CR programme has a fixed educational content, closed groups are run. There are pros and cons for each approach. A closed group allows the attendees to remain constant throughout, increasing the likelihood of shared experiences and group bonding or cohesion. Shared experiences are a vital part of the group process. Keeping the group closed enables people to feel more contained in sharing their experiences, thoughts or feelings. It also facilitates gathering together groups of patients who are at roughly the same stage of their recovery, enabling patients to identify with each other more easily.

Careful consideration has also been given to the ordering of the educational and the psychology talks within the CR programme. The talks complement each other as part of the multidisciplinary approach to cardiac rehabilitation. Having a fixed attendance allows the team to control the delivery of the talks in the preferred order.

Partners and family members are encouraged to attend the CR programme. Family or social support is an important part of the rehabilitation process. The CR team is available to provide support, advice and encouragement to family members or friends who are supporting the patient. This also helps to ensure that the rehabilitation messages are consistent, both at home and in the CR group. Retention of information is also likely to be increased with the attendance of a partner or friend, who may subsequently reinforce certain aspects of the programme.

Venues for CR

In order to reduce barriers to attendance wherever possible, all of the community venues in Gloucestershire are screened for patient accessibility and convenience. Adequate parking, proximity to public transport links and access to a telephone are essential requirements for each venue. Fundamental requirements for the room where CR is delivered include disabled access and toilets, adequate space for exercise, suitable chairs, presentation equipment (whiteboard or flipchart and pens), storage facilities for rehabilitation equipment and tea- and coffee-making equipment.

Health, Safety and Essential Equipment

The availability of resuscitation equipment is an essential aspect of a CR group programme. Each venue in Gloucestershire has a cardiac defibrillator that is checked at the beginning of each session. Other essential equipment includes a step for exercise, weights, exercise circuit pictures, heart-rate monitors, water jugs and cups. Models of the heart and of the coronary arteries can be useful teaching aids at CR groups if available. A regular standard health and safety assessment is carried out at each venue and the team members facilitating groups at the venue familiarise themselves with the relevant assessment.

Chapter 5

Coronary Heart Disease, Psychology and Exercise (Week 1)

Session Plan for Week 1

1. Introductions to the Cardiac Rehabilitation Programme (15 minutes)
2. Coronary Heart Disease and its Risk Factors (40 minutes)
3. The Psychological Side of a Cardiac Event (20 minutes)
   Tea and coffee break (15 minutes)
4. Goal-setting and Pacing (15 minutes)
5. Introducing the Exercise Programme (15 minutes)

Having made adequate preparation for beginning the programme (see Chapter 4) you are now all set for the patients (and their partners if partners have been invited to the programme) to arrive and for the first session to begin. The CR team normally arrive at least half an hour before the start of each session. This is to prepare for the session and to discuss individual patients. This is especially important before Week 1 so that the team can familiarise themselves with the diagnosis of individual patients.

As the attendees arrive at the venue and sit down, preferably in a semi-circle of seats, questionnaires that have been sent to patients can be collected and name badges given to both patients and their partners. Once all of the potential attendees have arrived and have been given a name badge, the first session can begin.

1. Introduction to the Cardiac Rehabilitation Programme

*The cardiac rehabilitation programme is introduced by one of the senior members of the CR team. The main points to be covered in the introduction can be written on the whiteboard before the patients and partners arrive so that they can be talked through by the team member introducing the programme (these main points are in **bold** below).*

The cardiac rehabilitation programme lasts for seven weeks and each session lasts for two hours. In the first session we will be introducing the programme to you and talking about coronary heart disease and its risk factors. We will also talk about why the psychological side of things is important in cardiac rehabilitation, and at the end of the session introduce the exercise programme. There is no exercise this week; the exercise programme will begin in the next session.

Before starting the main part of the session there are a number of introductions to be made, starting with the **team members** who will be on the cardiac rehabilitation programme for the next seven weeks (*introduce yourself and the team, mentioning their professions*).

A number of housekeeping items need to be mentioned before beginning the programme (*point out where the **toilets** and the **fire exits and assembly points** are in the particular venue*).

If anyone in the group has difficulty **hearing** then they might benefit from moving nearer the front of the group in order to hear better. The team will attempt to talk loudly and project their voices. Similarly if anyone is having difficulty in **seeing** what is written on the whiteboard then they may wish to move closer to the front of the group.

There are a number of **aims of the cardiac rehabilitation programme**. These are to provide information on coronary heart disease and its contributory factors and to help individuals to make the most of their recovery both physically and psychologically. This may involve making lifestyle changes. The interaction of the physical and psychological aspects of cardiac rehabilitation will be discussed in this session, and in future weeks the focus will be on lifestyle change and how to address the risk factors for coronary heart disease. At the end of this session today we will provide a **handbook/handout** that accompanies the programme/today's session and which will explain week by week what will be covered on the programme.

During the seven weeks of the programme the team will be referring to your **cardiac event**. By cardiac event we mean heart attack, coronary artery bypass graft (or CABG), angioplasty and stents, or angina. A cardiac event is the reason that individuals attend cardiac rehabilitation, and some people will have experienced more than one cardiac event. Rather than continually referring to "heart attack, coronary artery bypass graft, angioplasty or angina", we will use the term "cardiac event" to cover all of these. The cardiac nurse will be explaining more about the different cardiac events and how they relate to coronary heart disease later in this session.

Having introduced the team members and talked a little bit about the cardiac rehabilitation team's aims for the programme it is really beneficial for the team to hear one thing that each of you in the group would like to gain from cardiac rehabilitation. Some people find it difficult talking in groups so just introducing yourself to the team is fine. (*Start at one end of a row or of the semi-circle and go round each patient in turn. Listen to and thank each patient for their contribution.*)

It is always very helpful for the team to hear what you want to gain from the cardiac rehabilitation programme. It is also reassuring to hear that the kinds of thing that you are hoping to gain from cardiac rehabilitation are very much in line with the team's aims for the programme.

The cardiac rehabilitation team would like the next seven weeks to be inter-active and for the group to feel able to ask **questions** during each session. If the team is unable to answer a question then every effort will be made to find out the answer for the next session. The team will not necessarily be able to answer every question in this first session, however! Coronary heart disease and cardiac rehabilitation are big topics and will be covered in detail over the seven weeks of the programme, so some questions may be referred to later in the programme. The team will be available before each session starts, during the break, and after the end of each session to answer urgent questions. Sim-ilarly if there is a personal issue that you would like to discuss with a team member then they will also be available at those times.

There will be a break in the middle of each session for **tea and coffee**.

2. Coronary Heart Disease and its Risk Factors

First of all we are going to discuss coronary heart disease and its risk factors. During the introductions we mentioned your **cardiac event** and how on the cardiac rehabilitation programme we refer to a cardiac event as including heart attack, surgery, angioplasty and stents, angina, or any combination of these. One of the aims of cardiac rehabilitation is to help you to reduce your risk of having a further cardiac event or indeed any further problems with coronary heart disease. Once we have discussed what coronary heart disease is (appreciating that this may be revision for some people), we will look at the risk factors for coronary heart disease and why it is important to address these risk factors.

Coronary Heart Disease

Write "Coronary Heart Disease" on the whiteboard and draw a simple pic-ture of the heart on the whiteboard with coronary arteries clearly visible (Figure 5.1). To save time, and if there is room on the whiteboard, this can be done before the group members arrive at the start of the programme. A plastic model of the heart demonstrating the coronary arteries (if available) can be a useful teaching aid. Alternatively consider using laminated pictures.

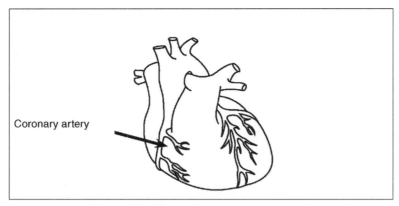

Figure 5.1 A heart, showing coronary artery

The heart is a muscle, about the size of your own clenched fist and it sits in the centre of the chest and a little to the left. Like any other muscle, the heart needs a good supply of blood containing oxygen and nutrients in order to pump efficiently, and it gets this through the coronary arteries. We have a left coronary artery and a right coronary artery. The left main coronary artery splits into two arteries as there is more muscle on the left side of the heart. The reason for this is that the left side of the heart is responsible for pumping blood around the whole body whereas the right side just sends blood to the lungs. The coronary arteries then split into lots of smaller arteries so that the whole of the heart muscle can receive a good blood supply. At birth these coronary arteries are smooth inside (*draw a cross-section of a clean coronary artery*) and have no "plaques" or "narrowings" or "furring up", and they provide a good supply of blood to the heart. Unfortunately, over a lengthy period of time these coronary arteries can become "furred up" (a process that can start in early adulthood for some people). The furring-up process involves fatty plaques being laid down in the walls of the coronary arteries. Initially you would not be aware that this process has occurred. Eventually, however, these fatty plaques can narrow the artery to such an extent (*draw narrowing of artery due to build up of fatty plaques*) that you may begin to experience symptoms of **angina**.

Angina

Write "Angina" on the whiteboard and draw a coronary artery with large plaque as in the example in Figure 5.2.

Angina is the name for the symptoms experienced when your heart muscle is not getting enough oxygen and blood to meet its requirements. Some of the group may have experienced angina whereas others may not.

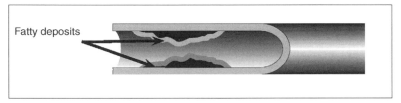

Figure 5.2 Plaque forming in coronary artery

If there is only a small amount of plaque in the coronary artery then enough blood will get through to the heart muscle (when at rest or when exercising) giving it the oxygen supply that it needs. In this instance no symptoms of angina will be experienced. However, when the plaques become larger, although enough blood can get through the narrowed artery when you are at rest, when you exercise your heart has to work harder to send more blood to the working muscles. Because the heart is working harder, it needs a better blood supply. If the increased blood supply cannot get through the narrowed artery then angina symptoms will be experienced. If you stop the exercise and rest, the symptoms of angina will go away. This is an example of what is called "stable angina". Stable angina can also occur when you feel stressed or anxious, because of the effects of adrenaline making your heart work faster.

Question to group: "Has anyone in the group experienced angina symptoms?"
Then: "What did the symptoms of angina feel like for you?"
Acknowledge the group's answers and emphasise how different the symptoms can be.

Angina symptoms are typically reported as a feeling of tightness, heaviness or pain in the chest, or other sensations in the arms, the throat or jaw. Some individuals report pain in the back or shoulders, while others report breathlessness as their main symptom of angina.

There can be many reasons for experiencing discomfort or pain or other sensations in the chest, arms, back, neck and throat. It is important therefore to get a diagnosis if you are experiencing symptoms. Some of the group may have undergone investigations such as a treadmill or exercise test, and/or an angiogram to investigate their symptoms.

Question to group: "Are any of these investigations familiar to you?"

The exercise test on the treadmill helps to confirm that you have coronary heart disease. This is done by working you hard over a short space of time to see if symptoms of angina are brought on by the exercise, or if any changes occur on the electro-cardiogram (ECG) to which you are attached.

During an angiogram, a very fine tube called a **catheter** is fed (through the groin) into an artery and up into an area where a dye can be injected into the coronary arteries. This dye will reveal (through X-ray) any fatty plaques in the coronary arteries. The doctor can then confirm if you have coronary heart disease.

Unfortunately there is no cure for coronary heart disease. It is, however, a condition that can be managed very effectively both through medical treatment and through moderating lifestyle to reduce the risk of any further problems. For some individuals the treatment can solely involve medication (and subsequent advice on how to moderate lifestyle) to help prevent any further build-up of these fatty plaques. For others it might be that the doctor decides that one or more of the narrowed coronary arteries requires opening with the aid of **angioplasty** and insertion of one or more **stents**.

Angioplasty and Stents

Write "Angioplasty and Stents" on the whiteboard. Draw a cross-section of a narrowed coronary artery with a build-up of fatty plaques. Actual stents, if available, can be a good visual aid. Consider laminated pictures showing the different stages of stent insertion as shown in the handbook.

Following an angiogram the doctor may decide to put one or more stents in the coronary artery/arteries as a treatment for coronary heart disease. This procedure may be performed immediately following the angiogram, or you may be asked to return at a later date to undergo the procedure. A stent is a tiny stainless steel mesh that is placed in the coronary artery to allow the artery to remain open and improve the blood supply to the heart muscle.

During the procedure to insert a stent, a catheter with a balloon on its tip is fed up into the narrowed coronary artery. This balloon is then inflated inside the narrowing of the artery so that the fatty plaque is squashed back into the wall of the coronary artery (*draw balloon inflated in the coronary artery and flattening the fatty plaques*). This will widen the narrowed artery and allow a much better blood and oxygen supply through to the heart muscle. This procedure is known as an **angioplasty**. Another catheter with a balloon and stent is then fed up into the artery. As this balloon is inflated, it places the stent into the artery. The area of narrowing is assessed so that the stent is the correct length and diameter for that artery; eventually it will become embedded in the artery wall (*draw a stent inside the coronary artery*). The stent then acts as a "scaffold" inside the artery keeping it open and allowing a good blood and oxygen supply through to the heart muscle.

For some people, depending on where the narrowing is in their coronary artery (and also how many arteries are significantly narrowed), the doctor may decide that a **coronary artery bypass graft** is the best way to manage their coronary heart disease.

Coronary Artery Bypass Graft (CABG)

Write "Coronary Artery Bypass Graft (CABG)" on the whiteboard. Show the group a plastic model of the heart demonstrating grafted arteries, if available. Consider a laminated picture demonstrating grafted arteries as shown in the handbook.

Like angioplasty and stenting, coronary artery bypass grafting, or CABG as it is known, is not a cure for coronary heart disease. It is, however, a very effective way of managing coronary heart disease and its symptoms. In a CABG operation the surgeon takes a vein or artery from the leg, arm or chest wall and joins it to the aorta in order to get a good blood supply. The new vein or artery is then grafted on to a point beyond the narrowed area in the coronary artery (*draw this on to the picture of the heart on the whiteboard*). The heart muscle below the narrowing will now receive a good blood and oxygen supply through this new blood vessel. The surgeon will graft as many arteries as necessary so this could be one, two, three or even four, depending on how many arteries are significantly narrowed. Most people who have had a CABG will no longer experience angina symptoms. However, it is very important after having a CABG to continue to manage coronary heart disease by taking medication and through living a healthy lifestyle.

Some people who have coronary heart disease may not experience any symptoms at all before having their cardiac event. It may be that they first become aware that they have coronary heart disease when they are taken to hospital having experienced a **heart attack**, or to give it its medical name, a myocardial infarction.

Heart Attack (or Myocardial Infarction)

Write "Heart Attack" on the whiteboard and draw a cross-section of a narrowed coronary artery.

When a person has a heart attack it is in most cases a symptom of coronary heart disease. A heart attack occurs when one of the fatty plaques in the coronary artery ruptures. It is not clear why the plaque ruptures when it does, and it is generally not related to what the individual was doing at the time of their heart

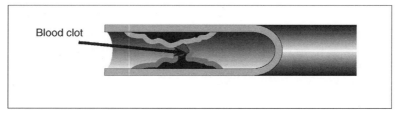

Figure 5.3 A clot blocks blood flow in the coronary artery

attack. The body recognises that there has been a plaque rupture and tries to seal it by sending clotting agents to the area. A blood clot then forms over the ruptured plaque, but unfortunately this can block the coronary artery so that no blood or oxygen is able to get to the area of heart muscle beyond the blood clot.

Draw the clot blocking the blood flow on the cross-section of the artery as in Figure 5.3. Outline on the simple drawing of the heart the area below the clot that would not be receiving any blood or oxygen as in Figure 5.4.

This part of the heart muscle may subsequently become damaged. Some people experience very few or no symptoms when having a heart attack. Others can experience (amongst other symptoms) chest pain or sensations in the chest or arms, nausea and sweating. Many people understandably are not aware that they are having a heart attack as the symptoms that they experience are not what they may have expected. Some people misinterpret heart attack symptoms as indigestion, as the sensation can be very similar to indigestion for some people. Others are expecting a heart attack to be just like it is portrayed on the television, that is, brought on in a stressful situation and accompanied by terrific pain! This is not most people's experience of having a heart attack.

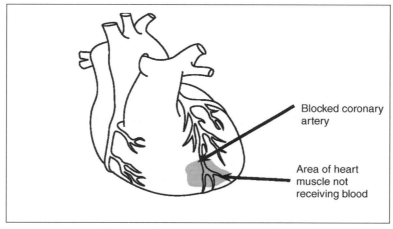

Figure 5.4 Damage to the heart muscle

> **Question to group: "What did having a heart attack feel like for you?"**
> *Acknowledge the experiences of the group.*

Some people delay getting to hospital because they are unsure of what is happening to them during a heart attack. It is important that an individual gets to hospital as quickly as possible, as there are different treatments available to treat the heart attack. These treatments aim to reopen the blocked artery, re-establish the blood flow to the heart muscle and thus minimise any damage to the muscle. Another reason for getting you to hospital quickly is so that we can monitor your heart rhythm and blood pressure.

If any patient has experienced a cardiac arrest it could be explained at this point.

One of these treatments is a clot-busting drug which can potentially dissolve the blood clot (thrombolysis). Sometimes it is very clear that a person is having a heart attack, from their ECG (heart tracing) and the discomfort that they are experiencing. In this instance the clot-busting treatment will be considered. This treatment, if given in the first few hours (and up to 12 hours after the attack), can disperse the blood clot and limit the amount of damage to the heart muscle. Clot-busting treatment is given through a vein and may have been given to you by the ambulance staff, in the accident and emergency department, or on the cardiac ward. For some patients who have been given an early diagnosis of a heart attack, an angioplasty and stenting may be the treatment of choice. This is the treatment we described earlier, and when performed at the time of a heart attack it is called primary angioplasty.

Sometimes after a heart attack there is an area of heart muscle that becomes permanently damaged. Over time it will become scar tissue, but the rest of the heart muscle carries on with the pumping of blood around the body. In the longer term exercise will be an important part of your rehabilitation, with benefits for your heart and the rest of your body.

If anyone in the group has been diagnosed with heart failure this condition could be explained at this point.

On other occasions it is not immediately clear that someone has had a heart attack, and a blood test is needed to confirm the diagnosis. It is possible that some of you were told one or two days after your hospital admission that you had a heart attack. After a heart attack was diagnosed your consultant may have requested further tests, which in most instances would have included an angiogram (and possibly a scan of the heart called an echocardiogram).

Following these investigations, some individuals would be prescribed medication and advice on lifestyle management, some may have an angioplasty and stent(s), while others may need to go on and have a coronary artery bypass graft.

So far we have discussed the symptoms of coronary heart disease, whether you experienced angina or a heart attack and the different ways in which coronary heart disease can be managed. It is now important to consider why the coronary arteries became "furred up" in the first place. To do this we need to look at the **risk factors** for coronary heart disease.

The Risk Factors for Coronary Heart Disease

Write "Risk Factors for Coronary Heart Disease" on the whiteboard.

The risk factors for coronary heart disease are a set of factors that make it more likely that coronary heart disease will develop in the coronary arteries. Some people with coronary heart disease will have a number of these risk factors while others may have only one or two risk factors. If we can take away or reduce some of the risk factors then in turn it will reduce the risk of developing further coronary heart disease and reduce the risk of further cardiac events. Most of the major risk factors for coronary heart disease will be discussed throughout the cardiac rehabilitation programme.

Question to group: "What are the risk factors for coronary heart disease?"

Or alternatively:

"What do you think caused one or more of your coronary arteries to become narrowed?"

Responses can be written on the board as in Figure 5.5. Make two lists under the headings of "Modifiable", or risk factors that can be changed, and "Non-modifiable", or risk factors that cannot be changed. When the lists are complete they can be discussed briefly, as most, though not all, of them will be discussed in more detail in future weeks on the CR programme.

The main risk factors for coronary heart disease can be divided into those risk factors that can be changed and those risk factors that cannot be changed.

The Risk Factors That Can Be Changed

These are the risk factors that we have some control over. If positive changes are made to these risk factors then it can lead to a reduction in the risk of developing further coronary heart disease.

Modifiable – things you can change	Non-modifiable
• Smoking • High cholesterol • Overweight • Lack of exercise • High blood pressure • Excess alcohol • Diabetes • Prolonged stress (links in with other risk factors)	Age Gender Family history Ethnic origin

Figure 5.5 Risk factors for coronary heart disease

Smoking is one of the main risk factors for coronary heart disease. It can cause damage to the inner wall of the arteries, raises blood pressure, reduces the amount of oxygen in the blood and affects cholesterol as well as increasing the stickiness of the blood. If someone continues to smoke after a cardiac event they are much more likely to go on to have another cardiac event. We will mention smoking on Week 4 of the programme. We know that although many people give up smoking at the time of their cardiac event others continue to smoke for a variety of reasons. There is a smoking cessation service in the county, and if anyone is contemplating giving up smoking then we can refer you on to that service for advice and support.

High cholesterol. Cholesterol is needed in the body. However, when we have too much cholesterol it can be deposited in the coronary arteries. We want cholesterol levels to be as low as possible following a cardiac event, and we will discuss cholesterol in more detail in Week 4 of the programme.

Being overweight is a risk factor for coronary heart disease, especially if the weight is carried round the middle of the body. It links in with high blood pressure and high cholesterol and also increases the risk of developing diabetes. We will discuss healthy eating in Week 5 of the CR programme as well as discussing the benefits of exercise for weight management. If weight management is one of your goals then we would advise you see your GP practice nurse for longer-term advice and support. There is usually a nurse in the GP practice who specialises in weight management. If this is not the case then we can refer you to one of the dieticians in the CR team.

Lack of exercise is a risk factor because your heart is a muscle, and like any muscle it needs to be exercised to function efficiently. It links in with other risk factors such as cholesterol and high blood pressure. We will talk about exercise each week as well as discussing the benefits of exercise in Week 6 of the CR programme.

High blood pressure over a long period of time has a direct effect on the heart muscle, the coronary arteries and other organs of the body. We will discuss high blood pressure in Week 3.

Alcohol becomes a risk factor when it is consumed in excess. It will be discussed along with healthy eating in Week 5.

Diabetes increases the risk of developing coronary heart disease. If diabetes is managed well, then the risk of coronary heart disease and other complications is reduced. It is important if you have diabetes that you are aware of what your target is for your blood sugar levels and the blood test HBA1c. Everyone who has diabetes should have a specialist nurse/consultant/practice nurse who can offer advice and support in managing this condition. If you feel you need more information please let us know and we can discuss this with you and refer you on as necessary.

Prolonged stress, or stress over a period of months or years, will be discussed in Week 2. Although not classified as a major risk factor, prolonged stress impacts on blood pressure as well as being linked to some of the other risk factors for coronary heart disease through the ways that we cope with stress.

The Risk Factors That Cannot Be Changed

Although these risk factors cannot be changed, it is important to acknowledge them as your risk factors. If any of them affect an individual then it becomes even more important to address those risk factors that *can* be changed.

Age is a risk factor, as the older that we get the more likely it is that we will have developed coronary heart disease.

Gender. Men develop coronary heart disease at a younger age than women. Women are usually protected by certain hormones until the menopause, but they catch up with men fairly quickly following the menopause.

Family history is important, particularly if a first-degree relative such as a parent developed coronary heart disease at a relatively young age—i.e. if the mother was below the age of 65 or the father was below the age of 55. If a parent develops coronary heart disease at a relatively young age, this can make it more likely that their children will develop coronary heart disease at a relatively young age too.

Ethnic origin. For a variety of reasons, coronary heart disease has been shown to be higher in individuals in the South Asian community in the UK.

During the course of the cardiac rehabilitation programme we will talk about these risk factors and how some of them are interlinked. For example, a person may experience prolonged stress, which they cope with by smoking cigarettes, which in turn pushes up their blood pressure. We will also discuss how to make lifestyle changes which can positively impact on one or more of these risk factors in Week 4.

In the handbook that accompanies this programme there is a section where you can identify your personal risk factors.

Risk factor information has been sourced from British Cardiac Society et al. (2005); British Heart Foundation (2004); and British Heart Foundation (2007a).

3. The Psychological Side of Having a Cardiac Event

We have looked at what happens physically when you have a cardiac event, but it is also important to consider the psychological side and how it relates to what has happened to you physically. By "psychological" we mean specifically how we think, feel and behave. Having a cardiac event can certainly have an effect on how you think, feel and behave as well as having a physical effect.

When people talk about what they would like to gain from cardiac rehabilitation they often say that they would like to become physically fitter or that they would like to return to certain activities and would like guidance on how to achieve this. However, there are other things that people may want from the cardiac rehabilitation programme. Regaining lost confidence or learning how to manage stress better are two of the commonly mentioned factors that are important to some (although not all) people after a cardiac event. They are also both feelings (and emotions), as we *feel* "stressed" and we *feel* confident or not so confident. On the cardiac rehabilitation programme we aim to help you with these feelings, and the thoughts and behaviours that go with them.

In fact, we are all thinking and feeling and behaving throughout each day. These are normal processes for all of us. (*Write "Thoughts", "Feelings" and "Behaviours" on the whiteboard as in Figure 5.6.*) Each of us also has a number of different physical responses every day, for instance our heart rate will go up and down or we may notice that we have a muscle ache in a particular part of our body (*add "Physical" to the whiteboard as in Figure 5.6*). Importantly, what we think about can affect how we feel and in turn this may affect what behaviours we engage in. As an example you may *think to* yourself "It's a lovely day outside – I'll go out for a walk". You might *feel* enthusiastic or motivated about this and so the *behaviour* that you engage in is to go for a walk (*demonstrate this on the white board while putting directional arrows on Figure 5.6*).

The physical effects from your body can influence this process as well. In the example on the board, feeling physically energetic encourages you to go for a walk. Conversely if, for instance, you had a bad cold it might be that although you are *thinking* it's a nice day to be going out for a walk you may

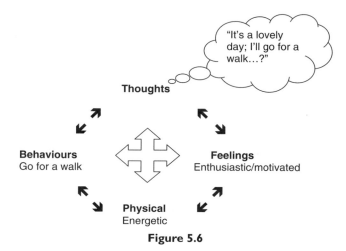

Figure 5.6

be *feeling* unenthusiastic about going because of the physical symptoms of the cold. Your *behaviour* may be that you end up going to bed rather than going out for a walk! Our thoughts, feelings, behaviours and physical sensations all have an effect on each other. Sometimes it is difficult to know which is affecting which. However, our thoughts, feelings, behaviours and physical sensations tend to work in cycles, which can be either positive or negative.

Thoughts, feelings, behaviours and physical reactions are therefore normal processes that we all experience every day. Following a cardiac event the impact on these thoughts, feelings and behaviours of the event itself will vary from individual to individual. It is certainly very normal, however, to feel some degree of stress or anxiety and to sometimes feel low in mood, especially in the early weeks following a cardiac event. As an example of how our thoughts in particular can be affected by a cardiac event (and how this can then affect your feelings and behaviours) we will consider the following scenario. Imagine yourself *before* your cardiac event sitting watching television and getting a sensation in the chest (*on the whiteboard figure, write "Chest Sensation" under "Physical"*).

Question to group: "What would you most likely think that the sensation was?"
Wait for the answer "Indigestion", and write it on the board as in Figure 5.7.

You would most likely *think* that the sensation before your cardiac event was indigestion.

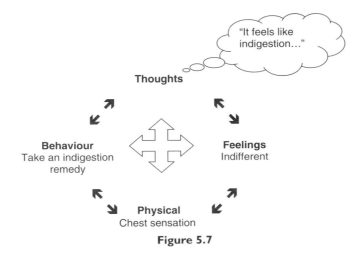

Figure 5.7

Question to group: "If you thought the chest sensation was indigestion how would that make you *feel*?"

Answers may be "Indifferent" or "Neutral", "Irritated" or "Annoyed" at the symptoms. Write them on the whiteboard under "Feelings".

You would most likely *feel* indifferent if you thought that the chest sensation was caused by indigestion.

Question to group: "In this situation what would your behaviour be? What would you do?"

Answers are generally along the lines of "Take an indigestion remedy"; write it on the whiteboard under "Behaviour".

You take an indigestion remedy and hopefully after a period of time, if indeed it was indigestion, the chest sensation would disappear. You would probably start thinking about something else or concentrate on the television programme you're watching.

Question to group: "So what if you had exactly the same chest sensation now? What would you be thinking?"

Answers are likely to be a variation on "Is it my heart?" Write answers on the whiteboard under "Thoughts" as in Figure 5.8.

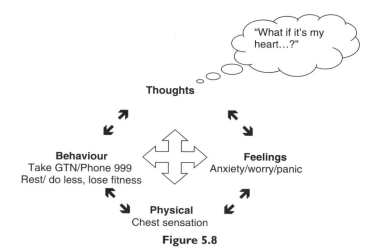

Figure 5.8

A normal thought following a cardiac event would be that the sensation might be related to your heart.

Question to group: "If you thought it might be your heart that's causing the sensation how would you be feeling?"
Answers are likely to be "Anxious", "Worried", "Stressed", "Panicked", "Frightened", etc. Write the answers on the whiteboard under "Feelings" as in Figure 5.8.

These would all be normal feelings if you thought that the chest sensation was related to your heart.

Question to group: "If you were thinking it was your heart that was causing the sensation and you were feeling some degree of anxiety, what would you do?"
Answers are likely to be "Take my GTN spray", "Phone 999", etc. Write them on the board under "Behaviour".

From the diagram on the board (Figure 5.8), it is evident that having a cardiac event can impact on our thoughts, feelings and behaviours.

The physical sensation in this example was the same as the one before we knew we had had a cardiac event. However, once we know we have had a cardiac event it is normal that we will interpret these kinds of sensations differently ("Is it my heart?"). In the example this has then led to different feelings (anxiety, stress) and different behaviours (GTN spray, phone 999).

Thoughts, feelings and behaviours will be discussed in more detail in Week 6 of the programme, in particular how our thoughts and feelings can sometimes prevent us from getting back to doing the things that we want to do following a cardiac event.

So this is the sort of psychology we will be covering on the programme. We are aiming to look at your recovery from both the physical and the psychological point of view so that you can make as much progress as possible. Traditionally, the medical profession has always been very good at patching you up physically and sending you on your way without always looking at the impact that an event has had upon you and your life. At this stage it can be helpful to think about what you have been through and the effect that it has upon you and the people in your life. It's sometimes reassuring to hear other group members report feeling the same things or having the same experiences. So in the last bit before a very well earned tea break, let's look at the impact that your cardiac event has had on you.

Question to group: "What have been the negative things about having had a cardiac event?"

Write down responses to the question on the whiteboard word for word under "Negatives". Responses will often cover the following.
Worrying thoughts:

- *How will it affect my life?*
- *How will it affect my partner/family?*
- *What if it happens again?*
- *What can I and can't I do at the moment?*
- *What about getting back to work?*
- *Will I ever get back to doing certain activities?*

Negative feelings:

- *Anxiety or panic*
- *Anger*
- *Irritability*
- *Frustration*
- *Feeling down or low*
- *Mood swings*

Being restricted in behaviours or desired activities is often mentioned, as well as "being wrapped in cotton wool" or being told by partners, families and friends to rest or not to undertake certain activities. Listen to, acknowledge and normalise these responses.

These are all normal thoughts, feelings and behaviours at this early stage after a cardiac event. It is common for partners to have these kinds of thoughts and feelings too. Often partners can be more anxious or worried than patients and may not want you to engage in certain behaviours because they are unsure of, or worried about, the consequences.

What about the positives?

Question to group: "Has anything positive come out of having a cardiac event?"

Some groups find it easier to come up with positives than others. Mention that it might seem an odd thing to ask at this stage but most groups will come up with a number of positives, whether they are positive thoughts, feelings or behaviours.

Responses to this question will often include that individuals now recognise what is important in life or that they no longer worry about little things. Other positives may be that relationships have become closer, friends and families have been supportive, medical care has been excellent or even the knowledge that having CHD is now an advantage in terms of "knowing what needs to be done" to manage it effectively. Write the responses on the whiteboard in the patients' words under "Positives". Some individuals may have experienced the exact opposite to the above and so it is important to mention that we are all individuals and will therefore respond to events differently.

We have seen that there can be positives as well as negatives after a cardiac event, and this is quite normal. One of our aims in cardiac rehabilitation is to help you to focus on some of the positive thoughts, feelings and behaviours after a cardiac event. We'll be talking more about positive and negative thoughts and feelings later in the programme.

Break for tea and coffee.

4. Goal-setting and Pacing

Still the psychologist speaking:

Goal-setting and pacing are twin concepts that run throughout cardiac rehabilitation. We will be returning to them frequently during the programme. At this stage of recovery there may be a number of things that you want to get back to doing. What is important is how you go about doing all of those things that you want to do.

The Problem: "Activity Cycling"

Question to group: "When you get up in the morning how do you decide what you are going to do on that day? What do you base your decision on?"
Responses to this question tend to include; the weather, work commitments, what's in the diary, how I feel, etc. Write answers on the whiteboard.

Most of us, at least from time to time, will base what we do on *how we feel*. There is potentially a problem, however, with basing our activities on how we feel. For instance, we might get up in the morning feeling good so we decide to go for a walk. We don't plan how far we're going to go as the weather's good (i.e. we'll just "see how we get on"), and we don't have anything else to do that day. Potentially we are at risk of overdoing our activity (*write this on the whiteboard as in Figure 5.9*) as we haven't planned how far we are going to walk (and unfortunately our bodies don't give us an early warning system to let us know that we are over-exerting ourselves). By the time we feel that we have done too much we have usually done *way* too much.

Question to group: "When we have overdone our activity how do we tend to feel?"
Responses will normally be "Tired", "Exhausted", etc. Write this on the whiteboard as in Figure 5.9.

When we're tired or exhausted we tend to rest (*write this on the board as in Figure 5.9*). We rest until we feel better, which can often be the next day, or in some cases a couple of days.

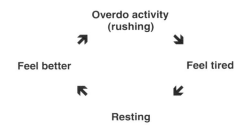

Figure 5.9 The "Activity Cyle" ("Rushing and Resting")

> **Question to group: "And then what do we do?"**
> *Responses are normally "Start all over again", "Overdo it again", etc.*

It can become a vicious cycle of "good days" and "bad days". Good days when we feel well and do lots of activities. Bad days when we are resting having overdone it on the good days! This vicious cycle is so common that it has its own name—the **"Activity Cycle"** (or sometimes it is known as **"Rushing and Resting"**). Once you begin to feel better, on a good day, the temptation is to rush around doing all the things you have left undone when you didn't feel like doing anything at all. It may be to mow the lawn, do the shopping or catch up with all the housework you've left undone. The problem is that we then tend to overdo it again in our eagerness to catch up, perpetuating the vicious cycle. Sometimes people will find themselves in this cycle from day to day so that they feel good in the morning but have to rest in the afternoon. This can lead to them labelling themselves as a "morning person". If we return to the Activity Cycle, it may be that they will wake up feeling good but because they have had recent experience of feeling exhausted in the afternoon they will then try and fit as much activity as possible into the morning as they know that they may need a rest in the afternoon! Often the very reason for their tiredness in the afternoon is because of overdoing their activity in the morning.

Over a period of time the problem with this vicious cycle is twofold:

1. It's difficult to plan your activity. It's hard to plan ahead because you don't know if you're going to have a good day or a bad day.
2. You experience periods of inactivity. This is when you are resting at the bottom of the Activity Cycle. The problem here is that when you are resting you will lose fitness. As a result when you get to the top of the cycle again you will be less fit than you were previously and will be able to achieve less before you need to rest again (*draw on the whiteboard as in Figure 5.10*). Gradually over the weeks and months you end up doing less not more (*draw on the whiteboard as in* Figure 5.10). This can lead to frustration, loss of confidence and ultimately disillusionment. It is common for people to stop doing activities if they are "activity cycling", as they may believe that they will never achieve what they would like to.

A cycle of rushing and resting is not an efficient way of doing anything. However, we know from experience that people who have had a cardiac event can make the most of their recovery and have the best chance of improving their fitness and stamina by using the simple principles of **goal-setting** and **pacing**.

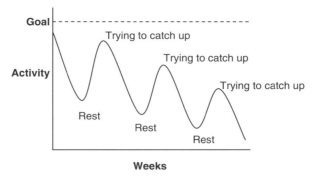

Figure 5.10 Diminishing returns from activity cycling

The Solution: Goal-setting and Pacing

The solution to the problem of overdoing our activity is to do things according to a plan, using a paced approach, rather than basing our activities on how we feel at any given time.

First we identify the activities that we want to be able to do more of. It could be walking, gardening, swimming, driving, housework, DIY—any activity that we may have reduced and that we now want to increase. These are our **goals**.

A useful way of thinking about how to achieve our goals is to use a goal-setting ladder (*draw a basic "ladder" on the whiteboard*). At the top of the ladder is our goal (*write "Goal" at the top of the ladder*). For each different goal we have a different ladder. The only way to the top is rung by rung. We need to break down our overall goal into mini-goals, with each one representing a rung. We need to plan ahead to some extent and to have thought about what each step will involve. This becomes clearer if we use an example. Our goal could be anything, such as getting back to doing the housework or cutting the lawn. We will use the example of walking a certain distance as this is something that most of us will be able to do. For this example the goal is to do a one-mile walk (*write this on the board at the top of the ladder next to "Goal"*). Some of us may never have walked a mile and others will be walking further than a mile even at this stage of recovery. It is, however, just an example and it is important to remember that everyone is an individual and therefore each person's goals will be different.

First of all it is necessary to discover the distance that we can always achieve, even on a bad day, which is not going to make us feel tired and need to rest. This could be walking to the corner shop and back, which might be, for instance, 200 metres. This becomes what we call our **baseline**, or the first rung at the bottom of the ladder (*write "Baseline" and "200 metres" on the board on the bottom rung*). The key to pacing ourselves effectively is that we will now walk to the corner shop every day (as we know that we can achieve this), but on the days when we feel good and believe that we could walk much further we *stick to this baseline level*. Once we are comfortable doing this every day it is time to step up to the next rung of the ladder. This could be walking to the paper shop and back (which might be, for instance, 300 metres), and so this becomes our new baseline. We would do this every day until we were comfortable and then we can step up to the next rung, and so on. Eventually, over a period of time, we will achieve our goal of walking a mile and will have done so without becoming trapped in the Activity Cycle of "rushing and resting". Rather than losing fitness and confidence by being forced to rest every few days, or every afternoon, we will experience a sense of achievement that we are working towards our goal. Our confidence should improve as we recognise what we are achieving with our activity, and our fitness will also begin to improve over time (*see Figure 5.11*). Ultimately we should feel more in control of our recovery. The important thing about goals is that when we have achieved them we can set ourselves some new ones if we want to!

Setting our goals in the first instance is important if we are going to achieve them effectively. We can have long-term goals such as "I want to be fitter", "I want to be myself again", or "I want to eat a healthier diet". These long-term goals need to be broken down into more specific goals such as "I want to walk a mile", "I want to be able to do my ironing" or "I want to eat five fruit and vegetables a day". It is then that we can consider our baseline and use the goal-setting ladder to pace our way towards achieving these specific goals.

Specific goals should also be realistic and achievable. It is better to set a number of easy goals and enjoy a lot of success rather than set really difficult ones that are going to take years to be achieved. If things don't go well, don't be discouraged. Think about what may have gone wrong and try something different. Writing our goals down and keeping a diary can help us to understand and focus on what we are trying to achieve (*see handbook/handout*).

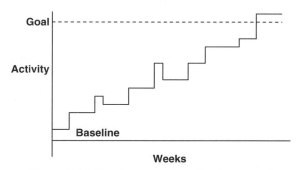

Figure 5.11 Paced progress from baseline to goal

Although it may sound easy, it can be very difficult for some people to pace themselves well. It is normal to want to finish what we have started, especially if it all seems to be going to plan. For example, we may be mowing the lawn and it's a beautiful day but we've already done our half-hour target and we are still feeling full of energy. It is very tempting to see how long we can carry on for, or carry on so that we get the whole of the lawn cut in one go. The problem of course is that if we carry on then we may well overdo our activity and slip into the cycle of rushing and resting. This can be especially common in the early days of our recovery when our baseline may be very low. It can seem unrewarding and frustrating to just weed 2 feet of a flower bed, paint one wall, or walk 50 yards. But this paced approach is the only sure and lasting way to recover fitness.

In summary:

1. Base what you do on a plan, not on how you feel, and keep to your agreed amount of activity. You will gain nothing by doing much more than you planned only to have to rest later or the next day as the result of exhaustion. This is the most common reason for not making progress.
2. If you are struggling generally, then it is probably because your baseline is set too high, so reduce it to what you can do more easily. Limit your activities if you are feeling unwell or have a heavy cold or the flu.
3. Increase your baseline at regular intervals (e.g. every week), even if it is only by a small amount.
4. Take all of your daily activities into consideration when thinking about setting your goals. Sometimes we can pace our exercise well but catch ourselves out by overdoing our housework, job or hobbies.

5. The Exercise Programme

Aim of the talk: to introduce patients to the practical exercise programme.
This talk is designed to give patients all of the information that they need to begin their practical exercise session in Week 2. Patients are initially introduced to the term "aerobic exercise" and asked to think about what types of exercise would be beneficial to their heart.

Question to group: "What kind of exercise will give the most benefit to your heart?"

Exercise

- Walking
- Cycling
- Swimming   **=AEROBIC**
- Dancing   **EXERCISE**
- Exercise classes

- Intensity-MODERATE
    ? Heart rate
    ? Breathlessness - telephone number test
    ? Exercise scale

Figure 5.12 Aerobic exercise

The answer is **aerobic exercise** (*write "aerobic exercise" on the white-board*). The word aerobic simply means "using oxygen" as a fuel. A useful way of understanding this is to use the example of going for a walk. As your leg muscles begin to work harder they will demand a greater blood supply. The heart begins to contract harder and faster so that it can pump blood to your working muscles. The working muscles then extract the oxygen they need from the blood stream. Just like putting petrol in a car to get it to run we need oxygen for our muscles to function!

Question to group: "Which particular exercises do you think are classified as aerobic exercises?"
Wait for the group responses and write on the whiteboard as in Figure 5.12.

Walking, cycling, swimming, dancing and exercise classes (at a moderate level) would all be classified as aerobic exercise. Aerobic exercise involves large movements of the arms and legs over a sustained period of time in order to build up the strength of the heart muscle.

Monitoring the Intensity of Exercise

When beginning an exercise programme there are a number of factors that need to be considered. Commonly patients will question how hard (with what intensity) they need to work when exercising. Ideally make this part of the session as interactive as possible, getting the patients' input on how they might know how hard they are working.

Question to group: "How do we know how hard we are working during exercise?"

This question will enable patients to consider some of the changes that occur in their body when they exercise.

The main ways in which we tend to know how hard we are working during exercise are:

- Our heart rate rises
- Our breathing rate increases
- We "feel different"

Write the above responses on the board.

Heart Rate

As we begin to exercise our heart rate will gradually increase. If our exercise reaches a fixed intensity our heart rate will then level off to a steady rate. An individual's resting heart rate and heart rate while exercising will vary depending on their age, their fitness level and sometimes on the medication that they are taking. We encourage patients to try monitoring their own heart rate while exercising at home over the coming week.

Tip: teach all patients how to find their pulse on their wrist or neck so that they can record their pulse when exercising at home.

Before starting the exercise session in Week 2, each patient should have an individual heart-rate training range calculated for them, using either the heart rate maximum or heart rate reserve method featured in Chapter 4. This should be done taking into account whether or not the patient is taking beta-blockers. Polar heart-rate monitors can be used during the practical exercise session for quick and easy monitoring of patients' heart rates.

Breathing Rate

During exercise it is normal for the rate and depth of our breathing to increase. Exercising at a moderate level should make us slightly out of breath but we should also still be able to hold a conversation.

The **telephone number test** is a simple test that can be used to estimate how hard we are working. During exercise it should be possible to say the whole of our telephone number, including the area code, in one breath without having to gasp in between.

Rate of Perceived Exertion/Exercise Scale

The Rate of Perceived Exertion (RPE) or Modified BORG Scale (see Figure 5.13 below) was developed in 1971. The RPE uses a 15-point scale rating from 6 to 20 with descriptions at every odd number. The scale has been shown to correlate highly with other variables such as heart rate, breathing rate and blood lactate concentrations. In the rehabilitation programme we tend to call this scale the Exercise Scale as this term is a bit more patient-friendly! Getting patients to use the scale correctly can initially be quite challenging. It is hoped that by the end of the cardiac rehabilitation programme they will have mastered the technique and will know what it feels like to be exercising at the right level for them. Patients are encouraged to use the Exercise Scale in conjunction with monitoring their heart rate.

Another way of monitoring how hard we are working during exercise is to use the Exercise Scale (*show the patients an example of the RPE*). While

6	**No exertion at all**
7	**Extremely light**
8	
9	**Very light**
10	
11	**Light**
12	
13	**Somewhat hard**
14	
15	**Hard (heavy)**
16	
17	**Very hard**
18	
19	**Extremely hard**
20	**Maximal exertion**

Source; Borg, 1998.

Figure 5.13 Modified BORG Scale

exercising you should choose a number on the scale that best represents how you are feeling at that time. You should give an *overall* rating of how you are feeling (including your breathing, how your muscles feel, any aching or other sensations). On the scale, 6 would be no exertion at all, so for example sitting quietly in a chair; 20 on the scale is the maximum exertion that we could possibly do, such as running up the side of Mount Everest with two bags of shopping!

Ideally patients should be encouraged to work between 12 and 13 on the scale, at a moderate intensity. However if you make this clear to patients in Week 1 they may subsequently always then tell you that this is the level that they are working at when you ask them during an exercise session! It is thus very important to highlight that it is their personal perception of exertion that is important to report.

Exercise Diaries

Ideally patients should be encouraged to fill out an exercise diary each week in order to keep a record of their exercise. If these exercise diaries are collected and read each week by the exercise professional it can be a useful way of spotting when a patient is overdoing their exercise. It is often not until the next day that patients realise that they have done too much.

Patients are encouraged to bring their CR handbook, with exercise diary, back with them each week so that they can talk individually with staff members about their current level of exercise.

Tips for Preparing for Exercise in Week 2

We will be starting the practical exercise in Week 2 of the programme and would advise you if possible to:

- Wear loose comfortable clothing
- Wear flat shoes
- Bring your GTN spray with you to the session
- Report any changes to your medication over the duration of the programme
- Report if you have experienced any symptoms in the last week
- Report any illness that you may have, e.g. a cold or flu

We would like you to arrive 10 minutes or so before the start of the session next week so that we can fit you with a heart-rate monitor. This will enable us to monitor your heart rate while you are exercising without having to take your pulse manually.

Any questions regarding the practical exercise session?

Chapter 6
Aerobic Exercise and Stress (Week 2)

Session Plan for Week 2

1. Exercise: What Sort and How Much? (10 minutes)
2. Exercise Practical (45 minutes)
   Tea and coffee break (15 minutes)
3. Stress and Coronary Heart Disease (50 minutes)

---

1. Exercise: What Sort and How Much?

Aim of the talk: to enable patients to think about the ideal type and amount of exercise that they should be doing following a cardiac event.

Session Set-up

Patients should arrive about 10 minutes before the start of the session to allow adequate time for the fitting of heart-rate monitors and to assess resting heart rates before the session begins.

The guidelines on exercise volume have been taken from the BACR Phase IV Training Manual (2006).

Exercise—What Sort and How Much?

The simple format in Figure 6.1 *below can be written on the whiteboard and used to explain the basic FITT principle of exercise. The answers can be left blank and then filled in if you choose to ask the group for their responses. The FITT principle gives a clear message about the ideal amount of exercise that is necessary to gain the greatest benefit to the heart.*

Welcome back to cardiac rehabilitation! Last week we talked briefly about how aerobic exercise at a moderate intensity would give us the most benefit to our hearts.

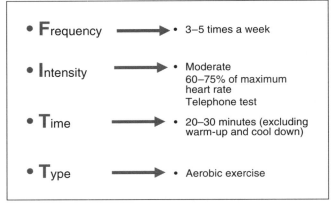

Figure 6.1 Exercise: what sort and how much?

Question to group: "How much aerobic exercise should we be doing each week?"

Each of the four parts of the FITT principle (e.g. Frequency) should be explained simply, giving the patients a clear message on how to build up their exercise. Reference should be made to the overarching principles of goal-setting and pacing discussed in Week 1. Patients are advised to start with the level of exercise that they are currently able to manage and to build their exercise up gradually over weeks and months in order to achieve their long-term goals.

Note. For some individuals; age, other conditions (e.g. stroke, arthritis or the severity of their heart condition) may mean that they will never be able to achieve the amount of exercise suggested. It is therefore important to highlight the benefits of even small increases in exercise. Even managing a small 10-minute walk every day is better than doing no exercise at all.

Question to group: "Do we recommend that you exercise every day?"

It is really what works best for each individual. If you can do some exercise every day then that is great as long as it fits in with the principles of pacing and goal-setting that we talked about in Week 1. It is important to keep the amount of exercise that we do each day to the same level so that we do not get into the cycle of "rushing and resting" that we talked about in Week 1.

Activity and Exercise

> **Question to group: "Does gardening count as part of your exercise?"**

Activities such as gardening and shopping are usually intermittent activities, and although they are beneficial to us they do not count as our aerobic exercise. This is because we might have periods when we are active and our heart rate is raised (e.g. when walking) but we will also have periods when our heart rate is lower (e.g. weeding or pruning). It is a common misconception that being generally active (e.g. gardening, shopping and housework) will give adequate benefit to our heart muscle. Typically activities such as housework are not sustained enough, or at a high enough intensity, to make them the aerobic (or cardiovascular) exercise that we talked about in Week 1 and which will increase the strength of our heart muscle.

I will illustrate this by drawing a diagram on the board (*draw* Figure 6.2 *on the board*).

The activity described in Graph A (gardening, housework) tends to be intermittent in nature. The graph shows how little time is spent in the training range. It is, however, important to recognise that what we all need in daily life is a balance between aerobic exercise and activity. Graph B shows how aerobic

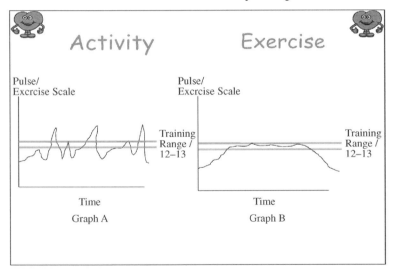

Graph A shows how intermittent activity may not be adequate enough to raise the heart rate for a continuous period of time
Graph B shows how with aerobic exercise the aim is to stay within the training range once the warm-up has been completed.

Figure 6.2 Activity versus exercise

exercise at the right level will keep an individual in their training range. It is this level of exercise that will give them the benefit of strengthening their heart muscle.

> **Question to group: "How fast do you need to walk to exercise your heart?"**

The pace that you walk at will be individual to you, depending on your fitness level. You should be able to say your telephone number (including the area code) out loud while walking, without gasping. You should never exercise if you have chest pain. Always rest and follow the protocol for the use of GTN spray if you experience chest pain while exercising.

It should be noted that we use a form of interval (rather than intermittent) exercise in cardiac rehabilitation classes. It is also important not to encourage complete rest during an exercise session as patients can be at risk of postural hypotension or arrhythmia due to sudden changes in their heart rate and blood pressure.

2. Exercise Practical

Following the talk a practical exercise session is held using a circuit format to allow individuals of different abilities to exercise together.

Break for tea and coffee.

3. Stress and Coronary Heart Disease

Stress management is an important part of managing coronary heart disease. Stress affects everyone, even if they are in good health, but following a cardiac event learning to manage stress becomes doubly important. In addition to the normal stress that we all have, after a cardiac event there is the added problem of coping with your recovery, which at times can be a source of stress in itself. The aims of this talk are to help you to understand what stress is, where it comes from, how it affects you, the link between stress and coronary heart disease and finally what you can do to manage stress effectively.

Prolonged Stress and Coronary Heart Disease

It is prolonged stress, or stress over a period of time (months, and in some cases years) that is linked with the development of coronary heart disease. This can appear contrary to our instincts, as we are often led to believe (especially through dramatic television reconstructions) that heart attacks in particular are more often than not "caused" by stressful experiences such as arguments or major shocks. Time after time on television we see a person having a major row and then clutching their chest and collapsing before being rushed to hospital having experienced a heart attack. Of course this will happen to some individuals, but you are as likely to have a heart attack in many other situations as you are during a heated argument.

In fact there are two main ways that stress is linked with the development of coronary heart disease. The first is that stress affects us physically and can increase our heart rate and increase our blood pressure. In some situations this can be a positive thing and can help to motivate us to do the things that we want to do. Over a *prolonged* period of time though, as we discovered in Week 1, stress becomes a risk factor for coronary heart disease and a potential trigger for angina.

Second, the ways that people have of coping with stress often actually increase their chances of developing coronary heart disease. For example when people are under prolonged stress they are more likely to smoke, drink alcohol, binge (or "comfort") eat, and take less exercise. In the same way that prolonged stress makes it more likely that we will develop heart disease, stress can also hinder our recovery. Good recovery in many instances involves changing enjoyable, well-established habits. These habits may have served us well in moments of stress, like having a cigarette while sitting in a traffic jam, or reaching for a cream cake or bar of chocolate. Prolonged stress makes it less likely that we will be able to maintain these changes.

Understanding Stress

Stress can be difficult to define in simple terms and often means different things to different people. We even have different words that we use to describe stress. For instance, some people will call it worry or anxiety rather than "stress". To understand stress we first need to look at the things which cause it. These we call the "stressors".

There are many different types of stressors and it is important to remember that everyone is different in the way that they perceive them. The things that you find make you feel tense or "stressed" may not have the same effect on another person. Something which may seem to be a stressor to you may not be for someone else.

> **Question to group: "What are the things that cause you to feel stressed?"**
> *Write the answers on the whiteboard under "Stressors".*

You should quickly develop a fairly long list of stressors often including things such as money, work, children, noise, neighbours, queues, driving and even marriage! It can help to use a prompt such as "What about the lists of the most stressful things that can happen to you in your life that you sometimes see in magazines or newspapers? What kinds of things tend to be on those lists?" It is also important to remind the group that they won't necessarily experience all of the stressors on the list, and in some cases may even find some of the things listed enjoyable. Driving is often cited as an example of this.

In order to understand the different types of stressors it is helpful to consider three broad groups. The first of these is **life events**. These are the one-off, big events that can cause us to feel stressed, such as moving house, getting married, divorced, etc. When you see lists of "the most stressful things that you will experience in your life", it is most likely to be such life events that appear on those lists.

The second group of stressors are known as **daily hassles**. These are the more ongoing daily, continuous sort of stressors, such as work, money worries or lack of time to do the things that you want or have to do. There tend to be a large number of these kinds of stressors in our lives (*go through the list of stressors on the whiteboard and point out the daily hassles*).

The third kind of stressors are known as **emergencies**. Emergency situations are single events which make us feel very stressed for a short period of time. Examples of these situations are an emergency stop in the car, or grabbing your child away from something very dangerous. These situations are less common for us and we tend not to have so many of them on our list of stressors. However, we will return to emergencies in due course as they show us something very important about stress.

Stressors can therefore be categorised into broad groups or types, and can be different for different people in terms of the effects that they can have. Stressors can be positive as well as negative, but most of all stress is an individual experience, and it arises through our interaction with our environment, whether that is through, for example, cars and our experience of driving or through people and our experience of our neighbours.

The Effects of Stress

> **Question to group: "How does stress affect us?"**

Stress tends to affect us in three different ways. It affects our emotions (or how we feel); it affects our thoughts or thinking; and, finally, stress affects us physically. In order that we can start to look at how we manage stress we need to examine how we are affected emotionally, physically and in our thinking in a bit more detail.

Emotions

Stress can affect people differently as we have seen, but if someone is experiencing stress then typically they may feel more frustrated, anxious, irritable, worried or tired. They may also feel tearful, low or depressed or find that they have lost their sense of humour. Feeling stressed for a prolonged period of time tends to drop our mood. When we are feeling low, life becomes harder to cope with and day-to-day things become more stressful. This can become a vicious circle.

Thinking

When experiencing stress a person may notice that their memory or concentration is not as good as it was. This is often the first thing that an individual will notice when they are under stress for any period of time. Often, though, they will not attribute these symptoms to stress and can worry that their poor memory or lack of concentration is being caused by something else, perhaps something more sinister. This can be another vicious cycle causing yet more stress. Negative thinking is much more common if you are feeling stressed (we will return to this in more detail in Week 6), and decision-making can become difficult.

People vary as to whether they feel the effects of stress emotionally or with regard to their thinking. Some individuals may find that both their thoughts and feelings are affected; for others, neither will be. But it is important to be aware that negative thoughts and feelings can be a sign that we are under stress.

The one reaction that we do all experience to stressors is the physical component.

Physical Effects

Physically we all tend to react in the same way to stress. To illustrate this we will return to the "emergency" stressors that we discussed earlier. These situations tend to show us the physical response to stress in an enhanced form.

I want you to imagine yourself leaving the building today and entering the car park, chatting to someone from the programme. You see a car driving much too fast coming straight towards you. You don't have time to get out of the way and you think that the car is going to hit you. At the last moment the car swerves out of the way and drives off.

Question to group: "What would you experience physically inside your body in this situation?"

Write responses on the whiteboard. Typically the responses will be "Heart rate increased", "Blood pressure increased", "Sweating" (palms especially), "Breathing fast and shallow", "Feeling sick" or "Butterflies in the stomach" and "Muscles tense".

There are about a dozen physical changes that occur altogether as a response to this kind of situation. These include your adrenaline levels going up and fatty acids being released into your bloodstream as a source of energy.

Taken altogether this collection of responses is what we call the "stress response" or the "fight or flight response", and it is caused by the release of adrenaline into your system (*write on whiteboard as in Figure 6.3*).

The stress response is in fact an ancient "life-saving" response that has been with us for thousands of years. In the dim and distant past this response was crucial to us as it prepared us to fight, run away or freeze, all of which were extremely useful to avoid or deal with an impending threat. The physical response involves muscles tensing ready for movement (indeed, ready to fight or run away). The heartbeat quickens to supply oxygen and other nutrients to the muscles and vital organs. Breathing becomes fast and shallow to supply the blood with much-needed oxygen. Blood is directed away from the extremities (such as the hands and feet) and the digestive system to the brain and major muscles.

In the present day the stress response can be very useful if we need to tackle a burglar or get out of the way of a speeding car, as it prepares us for action. The stress response is very noticeable in these types of emergency situation, but it is not where the link is with coronary heart disease. Our bodies are designed to deal with the stress response in these situations and will quickly return to

- Heart rate increased
- Blood pressure increased
- Sweating (especially palms)
- Breathing fast and shallow
- Feeling sick or butterflies in the stomach
- Muscles tense

Figure 6.3 The stress response (or "fight or flight" mechanism)

normal once the situation has passed. This does not therefore cause us problems in the longer term. To find the link with coronary heart disease we need to look at our daily hassles, as we also experience the stress response as a reaction to these day-to-day stressors. For example we can experience the stress response when we are frustrated by waiting in a long supermarket queue or when we are worrying about something. In these situations the stress response is at a much lower level but it is the same response. Unfortunately, though, the stress response is not useful in these situations. The body is getting geared up for action, but no physical response is actually needed. In effect our modern lives cause us to experience the stress response in a different way, but we have not yet evolved a new way of dealing with it. Over time this low-level response can gradually build up and start to cause symptoms. Some of these symptoms we may not necessarily relate to stress (such as loss of memory or concentration). It can push up our blood pressure, bring on angina and cause other physical changes, as well as changes to how we feel and to how we think. To cope with some of these changes we often find that we drink more alcohol, smoke more or eat more. We may also find it difficult to relax, or we may stop exercising, all of which are potential risk factors for coronary heart disease.

The Gradual Build-up of Stress

An average person's stress levels can build up over time, and typically as we go through life our stress levels rise. As we grow up and become young adults several things tend to occur. First, we typically experience a number of life events such as exams, leaving school, getting a boyfriend or girlfriend, getting our first job, getting married, having children and buying a house.

These life events are all stressful in themselves, but, importantly, two things occur as a result. First, they tend to bring with them a large number of daily hassles: in particular coping with work pressures and all the issues involved with bringing up children can be very stressful. What also tends to happen, particularly when we have children and start working, is that our time "shrinks". It may be that previously we used to have time to go out with friends, or play sport, or go to bingo or the cinema. We now find that we are getting home late from work or that all our time is taken up managing young children. Not surprisingly some of the hobbies and leisure activities that we used to enjoy don't seem possible any more, as we don't have time to fit them in.

As time goes by, then, typically these hobbies get left by the wayside. The problem is that these are often the very activities that have helped us to relax and cope with stress in the past. Furthermore, we tend to look for the "quick fix" that will help us cope with the long hours of work or stressful, busy days. So we may drink, smoke or eat more to cope with stress whereas previously we may have exercised or spent time relaxing doing the things that we enjoyed. Of course these "quick fixes" are generally less effective in helping us to cope with stress as well as also being risk factors for coronary heart disease.

Over time what we see is a gradual build-up of all aspects of the stress response. There is a build up in muscle tension, your heart rate and blood pressure can rise and your breathing can gradually become faster and shallower. This can all happen very gradually: most people don't realise that it is happening at all, and that they are becoming more physically tense. Our modern sedentary lifestyles don't help this process. In decades gone by we were much more active in and around the home as we didn't have all the modern "time-saving" devices that we have now. A housewife in the 1950s, doing her usual weekly housework, expended the same amount of calories as running a marathon! We are nowhere near as active as we should be, and this makes it harder for us to cope with stress. Our stress/tension levels can therefore continue to rise until eventually we reach a stage where we become aware of some of the symptoms (such as lack of concentration, headaches, sweats, poor memory, irritability, etc.).

Often, though, we do not relate these symptoms to stress. It is at this stage that little things tend to affect us in a big way. For instance we may become angry if someone says the wrong thing to us, or we may become tearful in situations that we would not previously have expected to. These are the kind of responses that you would not normally experience if your stress levels were lower.

When Stress becomes a Problem

We need a certain amount of stress to "get us going". If we never had any pressure to get things done we'd soon get listless and feel low. Life would be dull and boring. Research has shown that too little excitement can be as bad for our health as too much. Of course, the level of excitement that each of us needs is an individual thing. It's when things get so stressful that we feel that we are not coping well any more that life stops being enjoyable. So stress is generally not a problem for us unless it is very severe or is prolonged in nature. Having nothing in your life but work and worry, being unable to switch off from your responsibilities and never stopping to relax are problematic.

In summary, if we look at stress over a lifetime then typically when we are younger we tend to cope with stress well because we have more time to ourselves and we use it to do the things that we enjoy and that help us to relax. As we get older we take on more responsibilities, and with them comes an increase in day-to-day pressures. Because of these and our lack of time we often stop doing the things that previously helped us to cope with stress, and we replace them with more harmful coping strategies that can also be risk factors for coronary heart disease. Eventually we can reach a level of stress whereby we may feel unable to cope or we find that we are no longer enjoying life.

> **Question to group: "How can we manage stress more effectively?"**
>
> *Write answers on the whiteboard as in Figure 6.4.*

Managing Stress

The most important thing that we can do is to learn to manage stress effectively. Research has shown us that effective stress management reduces blood pressure and the risk of having another cardiac event.

The key to successful stress management is to focus on your "daily hassles". These can be relatively low-level, but they are important to manage, as we have seen how they can build up over time. How you cope with "life events" when they come along will depend to a certain extent on your background levels of stress (those caused by your daily hassles). Life events, or those one-off stressful times such as moving house, bereavement, a new job, weddings, etc., can sometimes be like buses, in that you might get a number of them together and at other times none at all. The key to coping with these situations is to have low levels of everyday stress so that you have the reserves to cope with life events if and when they come along.

Stress Management

The first step towards managing our stress levels is to **recognise our stressors**. Stressors will be different for different people, but becoming aware of our stressors is half the battle in terms of managing stress. Once we are aware of the causes of stress then we can start to address them.

> - Recognise our "stressors"
> - Regular exercise
> - Positive thinking
> - Change what can be changed
> - Time management
> - Talking about it
> - Learning to relax

Figure 6.4 Managing stress more effectively

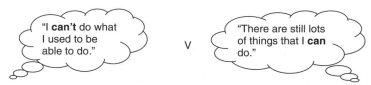

Figure 6.5 Negative thoughts versus positive thoughts

We have talked a lot already about **exercise**, and in Week 6 we will talk in detail about all of the benefits of regular exercise. Regular exercise is often described as a fantastic, "stress-buster" as endorphins are released into our blood stream while we exercise that help to make us feel good afterwards. Regular exercise also helps to lower our heart rate and blood pressure and improves our breathing, all of which are negatively influenced by the stress response. Exercise is therefore one of the best ways in which we can help to manage our stress levels. One of the other main benefits of exercise is that it helps us to relax more easily. At the end of this session we will look at relaxation and how we can learn to relax better.

Stress is caused through our interaction with our environment. It is therefore **how we perceive a situation** that is important in whether we find something stressful or not. One person may find a certain situation stressful (and feel that they do not have the resources to cope in that situation) whereas another person may find the same situation challenging, exciting and even enjoyable. Having to deliver a speech at a wedding would be an example of this. One person would relish such an opportunity whereas another would find it a very stressful experience indeed. Managing your thoughts in relation to a situation therefore becomes important in ultimately being able to control and reduce your stress levels. Thinking in a negative way – such as "I can't do this" or "If I do it, it will turn out to be a disaster" – will increase your stress levels. Unfortunately this kind of thinking can become a habit (you automatically think negatively) and it may be a habit that you have had for a very long time. It is, however, possible to change the way that you think about situations. Recognising when you are thinking in a negative way is the first step to **changing the way that you think** in these situations. It is then important to replace the negative, stress-inducing thoughts with a positive **stress-reducing** thought. Examples might be "I can do this" or "I can do this to the best of my ability and that will be good enough". Eventually if you practise this often enough it will become as automatic to think positively as it was previously to think negatively.

Changing what can be changed and accepting what cannot be changed is another important way for us to deal with our stressors. If we think more positively then we tend to feel more inclined and able to make changes to our environment, whether that is saying "no" to extra work, reducing our social commitments or reorganising our day to give us more time to relax. Generally, though, we have choices in life, and although there are some things we are not able to influence there are plenty of others that we can. By focusing on the things that we can change then we are able to positively influence our stress levels. Linked to this is the issue of **time management**. We often find that the reason that we are stressed is because we don't have enough time to do all the things that we need to do in a day. Sometimes we carry round in our heads an ever-increasing list of things to do which can eventually seem overwhelming. We subsequently end up doing none of the things on our list. We cannot create more hours in the day, but we can use those hours more effectively. Writing a list of the most important tasks and then prioritising these tasks in order of importance can be a very effective way of lowering our stress levels. Learning to "let go" of the less important tasks on our list until the next day (or sometimes for ever!) is part of the process of managing our time better.

Talking about how we feel is an effective way of managing stress for most of us. When we are stressed we can lose our perspective on life and get things out of proportion. Talking with friends or family can help us to regain our perspective on situations and become more positive in our thinking. We will return to this in Week 5 when we talk about how to make the most of your recovery.

Finally we know that **learning to relax** well will definitely help us to lower our stress levels. Relaxation is a skill, but unfortunately it is a skill that many of us are not particularly good at! However we can *learn* to be better at relaxation, and over the next few weeks we will focus on different ways in which you can learn, with practice, to relax more effectively. There are many benefits of relaxation. When we are relaxed we cope better with our stressors (whether that is work, looking after children, or being a carer), we find it easier to exercise, we tend to sleep better, our blood pressure reduces, we feel less tension and our mood improves. We will start with a very simple but effective method of relaxation known as abdominal breathing (sometimes known as "diaphragmatic" breathing).

Abdominal Breathing

Abdominal breathing is the most simple and easy-to-use relaxation technique of all, and because of this it is the most useful. It is simply a form of deep breathing. With a bit of practice abdominal breathing can be done at any time and in any place. Abdominal breathing, when practised on a regular basis, is important for the three reasons shown in Figure 6.6.

1. Your breathing and your heart rate are affected by the stress response, so it is important that they are controlled. Abdominal breathing helps you to do this.

2. Abdominal breathing enables you to tense and relax all the major muscles in the top half of the body. This sequence of tensing and relaxing muscles is a useful form of relaxation in itself (as we shall see later in the programme).

3. Developing abdominal breathing as a habit is a good way of reminding yourself to pay attention to what your body is doing on a regular basis and so will help you to monitor your stress levels.

Figure 6.6 Why is abdominal breathing important?

Practising Abdominal Breathing

Àbdominal breathing means using the diaphragm, the sheaf of muscle under the lungs, and the abdominal or tummy muscles. What should happen when you take a slow deep breath in is that as your lungs fill with air, the diaphragm pulls down to help them expand and take in lots of oxygen. As a result of this your stomach should swell out as you breathe in. Some people find that when they try this it feels strange as they are used to their stomach moving in when they take a breath. However, that is very much a "tensing" breath and not a relaxing one. When we breathe abdominally our nervous system does exactly the opposite of what it does during the stress response, helping us to feel relaxed. It can be difficult and unusual to breathe abdominally at first, and it is a good idea to practise when possible. With practice, it will become easier over time.

To breathe abdominally while sitting you should make sure that you are sitting upright on the edge of your chair. Make sure that you are comfortable and put your right hand lightly on your stomach with your little finger just above your belly-button, resting your left hand above it on your chest. Taking a slightly deeper than normal breath, push your stomach out as you breathe in through your nose. As you do this, look at your right hand, it should move as your stomach moves. If this happens, it means that you are using your diaphragm to breathe. If you do not get any movement then your breathing is all coming from your chest. This will make you *more tense* in the longer term. Breathe out slowly through your mouth (*practise a couple of abdominal breaths with the group*).

Some people find it quite difficult to breathe abdominally to begin with as they are used to breathing from their chest. Ideally you should practice this technique regularly and to build up a routine of taking one or two abdominal breaths every half an hour (so that you are doing 20 or 30 abdominal breaths every day). It will become easier and more effective over time. To help you to remember to practise your breaths we have devised a monitoring system for you using self-adhesive coloured dots! (*Hand out half a dozen coloured dots to each individual.*) The idea is to take these home and stick them wherever you will see them during a typical day: on the kettle, the radio, the TV remote control, your watch, or the steering wheel of your car. Every time that you see a red dot during the day do a couple of the abdominal breaths. You can also think to yourself, "How am I breathing? Is it shallow and quick, and do I need to do a couple of abdominal breaths?" This way you will get into the habit of becoming aware of what your breathing is like throughout the day, and you will also get into the habit of doing a couple of relaxing breaths every half an hour or so. Do not do more than two breaths at a time as you may feel light-headed due to the increased amount of oxygen that is in your system when breathing abdominally. However if you practise it regularly it will have the effect of making you feel more relaxed from day to day as well as being a very useful management tool to use in stressful situations. We will ask you how you are getting on with your abdominal breathing in a couple of weeks' time.

Information on stress as a risk factor in this chapter has been taken from Bunker et al. (2003) and British Heart Foundation (2004).

Chapter 7

Warming Up, Cooling Down, Angina and Hypertension (Week 3)

Session Plan for Week 3

1. Warm Up and Cool Down (10 minutes)
2. Exercise Practical (45 minutes)
   Tea and coffee break (15 minutes)
3. Angina (30 minutes)
4. High Blood Pressure (20 minutes)

---

1. Warm up And Cool Down

Aim of the talk: to introduce patients to the idea that a thorough warm-up and cool-down is important in allowing safe and effective exercise.

Warming up

This talk should be as interactive as possible, asking individuals to think about the possible reasons for doing a warm-up before exercise.

Question to group: "Do you think that it is a good idea for us to get up (e.g. out of a chair) and set off at our normal walking pace?"

Figure 7.1 shows how this talk can be structured by first getting patients to give the reasons for warming up and then writing them on the whiteboard. Each point in Figure 7.1 can be expanded upon to give patients the reasons behind doing a proper warm-up.

- Why?
    - Gradual increase in heart rate and blood pressure
    - Increased circulation to working muscles
    - Increased breathing rate
    - Coronary arteries dilate, allowing extra blood flow to the heart muscle
        - Less chance of getting angina
        - Allows greater duration of exercise session
    - Reduces injury risk
    - Psychologically prepare for exercise
- How long for?
    - 15 minutes

Figure 7.1 Warm up

Heart-rate elevation

As our muscles begin to work harder during exercise they demand more oxygen. This is achieved by speeding up the heart rate in order to pump blood around the body faster. We need this to happen gradually so that our body has got time to make these changes.

Blood-pressure elevation

It is normal for our blood pressure to rise during exercise and it will go back down to normal (or even lower) when our exercise session is finished.

A gradual warm-up means that our blood pressure will rise gradually (rather than suddenly) giving time for our body to cope with the change.

Increased circulation

Oxygen is carried in the bloodstream. The muscles being used during exercise will need a better blood supply to get the increased oxygen that they need while exercising. This is achieved by the dilation of blood vessels in the working muscles and also the gradual increase in heart rate.

Increased breathing rate

In order to get more oxygen into the body during exercise we breathe faster and deeper. It is perfectly normal to be a little out of breath during exercise (*refer to normal scores for RPE scale for warm-up, i.e. 9–10*).

Coronary artery dilation

If the heart is working harder (as it is beating more often) it also needs a better blood supply via the coronary arteries. Our coronary arteries are able to dilate over time and allow a greater blood flow through them.

Reducing angina   If the coronary arteries have time to dilate there is less chance of someone getting angina symptoms. This can often mean that an individual will be able to exercise for longer.

Reduced injury risk   As the circulation to the working muscles speeds up they get warmer and become more flexible, allowing a greater range of movement, reducing the risk of straining or tearing a muscle.

Mentally prepare   Warming up will gradually increase the adrenaline levels in the bloodstream, which in turn will increase our level of alertness.

Question to group: "For how long should we warm up?"

We should be warming up for 15 minutes. It takes that long for our coronary arteries to dilate properly and for our muscles and circulation to respond effectively.

Types of Warm-up Activity

Question to group: "What types of activity can we do to warm up?"
Responses can be written on the board, as in Figure 7.2 .

A warm-up can be as simple as starting off walking at a slower pace than normal and then gradually building it up over a period of 15 minutes. You may also choose to do a structured warm-up similar to the warm-up exercises that you complete during the cardiac rehabilitation exercise session.

- Walking slowly on the flat and gradually building up the pace
- Walking around the house before going outside on a cold day
- Using a structured warm-up routine, e.g. marching on the spot, shoulder rolls, stretches
- Cycling on the flat in a low gear

Figure 7.2 Types of warm-up activity

- Why?
  - To reduce the heart rate and blood pressure slowly
    - Avoid feeling dizzy due to a sudden drop in blood pressure/heart rate
  - Coronary arteries go back to their normal size
  - Reduce circulation gradually
    - Get rid of lactic acid
    - Reduce injury risk
- How long?
  - 10 minutes

Figure 7.3 Cool down

Cooling Down

Cooling the body down after exercise is just as important as warming up. Stopping exercise suddenly can be problematic especially if you have had a cardiac event.

Question to group: "Why do we need to cool down?"
Responses can be written on the board, as in Figure 7.3 .

Each point in Figure 7.3 can be expanded upon to give patients the reasons behind doing a cool-down.

Heart rate reduces	It is important to avoid any sudden changes in our heart rate following exercise as it can potentially cause abnormal heart rhythms to occur.
Blood pressure reduces	Going from exercise to rest in a short space of time can cause our blood pressure to drop suddenly, leaving us at the risk of hypotension (low blood pressure) and as a result possibly feeling faint or light-headed. This is because the muscles in our legs (especially the calf muscles) are responsible for helping to pump blood back to the heart against gravity. If exercise is stopped suddenly, the leg muscles stop pumping the blood back to the heart, causing a reduced blood supply to the heart and the head.

Circulation   Sometimes during exercise lactic acid can build up in our muscles, and if it is not removed it can cause our muscles to ache the next day. With a gradual cool-down our circulation can help to get rid of that lactic acid so that our muscles don't ache the following day. It is also important to stretch our muscles following exercise as this helps to reduce the risk of injury.

Ideally patients should be close to their resting heart rate at the end of the cool down. However, some individuals may need longer for their heart rate to return to its resting rate. Their recovery rate may improve with time as their fitness level improves. A faster heart-rate recovery can be an indicator of improved fitness. Older people tend to have a slower baroreceptor reflex (responsiveness to changes in blood pressure) and therefore may need longer than 10 minutes to cool down.

How do we Cool Down?

Question to group: "What types of activity can we do to cool down?"
Responses can be written on the board, as in Figure 7.4.

Stretching

Encouraging the use of stretching in the warm-up and cool-down is important. Stretches should be held for about 10–15 seconds (up to 30 seconds during the cool-down) ensuring that patients do not hold their breath during the stretch (as this will increase their blood pressure). Of particular importance are the chest and shoulder stretches for individuals who have had bypass or valve surgery, as there may be risk of muscles shortening following the surgery.

Proprioceptive neuromuscular facilitation (PNF) stretches should be avoided in this population group due to the static muscle contractions that are used with this technique.

- Walking slowly on the flat at the end of an exercise session
- Doing structured cool down exercises and stretches
- Cycling slowly in a low gear

Figure 7.4 Types of cool-down activity

2. Exercise Practical

Following the talk a practical exercise session is held using a circuit format to allow individuals of different abilities to work together.

Break for tea and coffee..

3. Angina

For this session a plastic model of the heart with the coronary arteries showing can be a good visual aid. Also a model of the coronary arteries showing progressive narrowing of the arteries can be used, along with a picture showing the process of stent insertion.

Draw a cross-section of a coronary artery on the whiteboard, showing fatty plaques (see Figure 5.2 above).

Angina is a symptom of coronary heart disease. In this session we will discuss what angina is, what angina feels like and what we can do about it. Some people in the group may not have experienced angina, whereas others may still be experiencing it. We talk about angina in order to help those who are having angina to manage their symptoms as well as possible, and also to help us recognise the symptoms if we were to have angina in the future.

What is Angina?

The heart receives its blood and oxygen supply through the coronary arteries. When we are born our coronary arteries have no "narrowings" or "plaques" so our heart muscle is always able to receive a good blood supply, whether we are at rest or exerting ourselves. For the reasons we talked about in Week 1, when we discussed coronary heart disease and its risk factors, over time fatty plaques can get laid down in one or more of the coronary arteries, causing them to become "furred up" and narrowed. This process can take many years, and it is only when the arteries are sufficiently narrowed that a person may experience symptoms of angina (*show the model, if available, of progressive furring up of the coronary arteries*).

Typically a person may not experience any symptoms of angina when resting because enough blood is getting through the narrowed arteries. However, when they are exercising, the working leg muscles need a better blood supply so the heart works harder and faster to supply the blood. Because the heart is working harder it too needs an increased blood supply, and if this blood cannot get through the narrowed coronary arteries then angina symptoms can be experienced. Usually, if we stop and rest the symptoms will go away.

> **Question to group: "Has anybody experienced angina in this way?"**

This is a common scenario and it is known as *stable angina*. This is when angina comes on with exertion and goes away again at rest. Although the symptoms are not pleasant, the heart is not damaged in stable angina.

Symptoms of Angina

It can sometimes be very difficult to differentiate between angina symptoms and other problems such as indigestion or musculo-skeletal problems. There are, however, certain things that can help a doctor make a diagnosis of angina.

> **Question to group: "For those of you who have experienced angina, what kind of symptoms did you have?"**
> *Acknowledge the different symptoms the group has experienced, thus highlighting how it can be difficult to make a diagnosis.*

The symptoms of angina vary from person to person, but common symptoms can include discomfort or pain, an ache or tightness, heaviness or pressure, a burning sensation, or even feeling short of breath. These symptoms can be felt in the chest area, across the shoulders or back, in one or both arms, in the neck, throat or jaw, or across the upper abdomen. Some people experience angina as breathlessness (more than they would expect to experience when they are exercising or exerting themselves). Some people will experience several of these symptoms, whereas others may just experience one. If you are experiencing symptoms for the first time or your existing symptoms are getting worse or more severe, then it is a good idea to keep a diary of the type of discomfort or pain that you are experiencing. It is worth noting what you were doing at the time, how long the symptoms lasted and what you did about them. You should make an appointment with your doctor to discuss the symptoms. The diary can help you and your doctor to decide if the symptoms may be angina. The doctor can then refer you to the hospital for further tests to confirm if it is angina or not.

Treatment for Angina

For patients who it is thought may be having angina, investigations such as an exercise test or an angiogram may have been requested to try and confirm the diagnosis. Following these investigations, if angina (and coronary heart disease) has been confirmed, the consultant will decide the best way to manage the condition. For some of you it might have been that the treatment to manage your angina was to be prescribed medication, along with advice on how to lead a healthy lifestyle. Others may have needed an angioplasty and the insertion of one or more stents.

Show the group a model of a stent and a picture of the process of stent insertion if available.

When the angioplasty is performed a catheter with a deflated ballon at its end is inserted into the artery. The fatty plaque that is causing the narrowing in the artery is squashed back against and into the artery wall by the inflated balloon. The stent is then inserted in order to hold the artery open so that a good blood supply can get through to the heart muscle. In most cases this will lead to a reduction in the symptoms of angina, and the majority of people who have a stent fitted will then be symptom-free.

For other people, depending on how many narrowings they have, or because of where the narrowings are situated in (one or more of) their coronary arteries, it may be that a coronary artery bypass graft (CABG) is the treatment of choice. In a CABG operation, arteries or veins from other parts of the body are taken and joined to a good blood supply (such as at the aorta) and also at a place beyond the narrowing. This is so that the blood supply can literally "bypass" the narrowing and feed the heart muscle below with a good supply of blood and oxygen. The narrowed artery is left in place and, because it is being bypassed, angina symptoms are reduced.

Following both stent insertion and CABG, taking medication and leading a healthy lifestyle will be important aspects in managing coronary heart disease in the longer term.

So far we have discussed what angina is; how it can be experienced differently from one person to another; how it is diagnosed; and the treatments that may follow a diagnosis. Following a cardiac event most people do not experience any symptoms of angina. This can be due to the medications prescribed or the interventions that they have had. However, others may continue to experience symptoms of angina, and it is important to manage these symptoms as well as possible.

Triggers for Angina

Triggers are the things that can bring on symptoms of angina.

Write the triggers on the whiteboard and then discuss more fully—see Figure 7.5.

- Exercise/exertion
- Being in a stressful situation
- Extremes of temperature – particularly cold weather
- Heavy meals

Figure 7.5 Triggers for angina

There are a number of common triggers for angina (*in bold below*). We have already mentioned that **exercise or exertion** can bring on symptoms of angina, so running for a bus or mowing the lawn would be examples of occasions when angina could be triggered through exertion. **Stress or anxiety** can also be triggers for angina. When we are stressed or anxious, adrenaline is released into our system, causing our heart to beat faster. When our heart beats faster it requires a better **blood supply**. If the coronary arteries through which it receives that blood supply are narrowed, it will not get the improved blood supply it needs, giving rise to the symptoms of angina. For some people **cold weather** can be a trigger for angina. A less common trigger for angina is a **heavy meal**.

So having recognised the triggers for angina it is important that we manage it effectively.

Managing Angina

There are a number of things that we can do to help us to manage angina effectively.

Question to group: **"What might help us manage angina effectively?"**

Exercise (and the Timing of Meals)

We know that angina can be triggered by exercise. However, if we *warm up* before exercising then the coronary arteries will open up and give the heart a better blood supply, preparing it for exercise and thus reducing the chances of experiencing angina. We do not want people to be exercising following a meal, as both the working muscles and the digestive system will require an increased blood supply, and this may bring on angina symptoms for some people. Following a light meal, we would recommend that you leave exercising for at least an hour. Following a heavy meal, we would suggest that you do not exercise for at least two hours, allowing plenty of time for food to be digested.

If we exercise regularly, however, we can increase the strength of our heart muscle so that over time our heart works more efficiently and is able to provide a really good supply of blood and oxygen to the working muscles without having to work so hard itself. This will mean that, over time, as our heart gets increasingly stronger, we can exercise for longer and longer before symptoms of angina occur.

For example, it might be that a person walks to a certain point every day, where they find that they have to stop because they are experiencing angina (*you can draw a simple diagram with a stick person walking up a hill to illustrate this*).

This might put them off exercising completely as they do not want to get angina (and, quite understandably, they think that if they do not exercise they will not get angina). The problem is that if they do not exercise they will also lose fitness, their heart will become less efficient and they are at risk of experiencing angina with even less exertion, or exercise, than at present. The best way to manage this situation is for the person to stop at a point before they experience their angina and to return home (*show this on the diagram*). If they do this every day, then over time, as their heart becomes stronger and more efficient because of the regular exercise, they will be able to increase the distance that they walk without experiencing any symptoms. Eventually they will pass the point where they were originally experiencing angina (we call this increasing their **angina threshold**). Using the principles of **goal-setting** and **pacing** that we talked about in Week 1, they can then decide on how far they want to walk in the future, hopefully without experiencing any further symptoms.

Stressful Situations

> **Question to group: "If you found that you were experiencing angina in a stressful situation what would you do?"**

Taking yourself away from a stressful situation, where possible, is an important and effective strategy in managing angina. Furthermore, abdominal breathing (discussed in Week 2) slows down the effect of adrenaline, lowering the heart rate as well as supplying the body with a rich supply of oxygen. A couple of deep abdominal breaths in a stressful situation can also help to manage angina. More generally, we all need to try and manage our "background" stress levels well by using some of the strategies that we talked about in Week 2, including regular abdominal breathing and relaxation. Next week we will be giving you a CD with three different relaxation techniques, which, if practised regularly, can help with relaxation. In particular the third technique on the CD, called Autogenic Relaxation, which improves your circulation, has been shown to be effective in helping to manage angina.

Cold Weather

If the cold weather brings on your symptoms of angina it is recommended that you wrap up warmly before you go out and consider using a scarf over your nose and mouth. Also consider doing the warm-up indoors.

If angina symptoms continue despite the above strategies then we would advise you see your GP so he or she can review whether further medication could help or if more tests are required.

What Do You Do if You Are Having Angina?

Most, if not all of you, will have been given a GTN (glyceryl trinitrate) spray, although some of you may have been given nitrate tablets instead. The GTN spray relaxes the coronary arteries, opening them up and therefore quickly improving the blood supply to the heart. If a person is having symptoms of angina then a spray of GTN under the tongue will often take away the symptoms very quickly. GTN spray can occasionally make a person feel light-headed, so it is advisable to sit down when using it. It can also leave some people with a headache after use.

> **Question to group: "If you were exercising and you experienced symptoms that you thought might be angina, what would you do?"**

The first thing to do is to **stop** what you are doing and **sit down** if possible. The most important thing is not to ignore any symptoms. If you have been exercising then you should keep your feet moving. Taking a couple of abdominal breaths can be helpful, and some people will find that this alone can take away their symptoms. If the symptoms continue then you should use your GTN spray if you have it with you (remember that if it is angina then stopping and resting will eventually relieve the symptoms, so there is no need to worry if you have forgotten your spray). The protocol for using GTN spray is as follows (*write the GTN protocol on the whiteboard as in Figure 7.6*).

The GTN protocol is adapted from the protocol included in British Heart Foundation (2006).

If the symptoms have not gone after 15 minutes then it is important that you are seen in hospital to determine the cause of the symptoms. It does not necessarily mean that you are having a heart attack, but it is important to find out what is causing the symptoms.

Question to group: "Would everyone be happy to use the protocol that we have just discussed?"
Acknowledge the group's responses, trying to determine if you think anyone would be hesitant to use the protocol. Discuss further as necessary.

If angina symptoms last for 15 minutes and you have rested and used the spray, we want you to call for help by ringing 999 and tell the operator that you have coronary heart disease. The ambulance service, GPs and cardiologists have agreed this protocol and want you to use it.

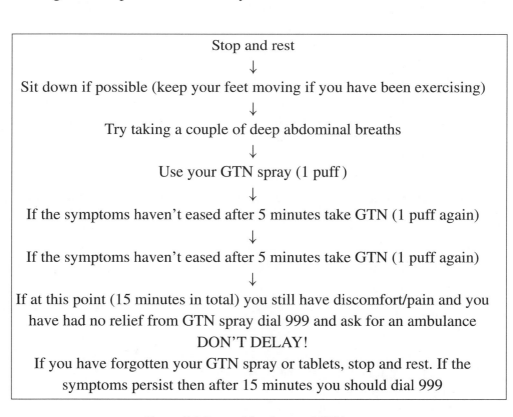

Figure 7.6 Protocol for the use of GTN spray

If you have not experienced symptoms of angina for months (or even years) and then in one week you have two episodes of symptoms that were relieved within 10 minutes, we would advise that you see your GP. This is so that he or she can review your medication and decide whether you need to be referred back to the hospital for further investigation.

Key messages:

- Explaining that angina does not damage the heart, thus reducing anxiety about angina
- Common symptoms of angina: how to know if it might be angina that you are experiencing
- Triggers for angina
- Self-management strategies: how not to be at the mercy of your symptoms, breathing, GTN, pacing
- Clarification of the GTN Protocol: when to seek help

---

4. High Blood Pressure (Hypertension)

For the final part of this session we are going to talk about high blood pressure (or hypertension). In Week 1, we discussed the fact that high blood pressure is one of the risk factors for coronary heart disease. High blood pressure is also linked to other conditions.

Question to group: "What medical conditions can be caused by having high blood pressure over a long period of time?"
List these conditions on the whiteboard: CHD, stroke, kidney damage, enlarged heart, heart failure.

High blood pressure over a long period of time increases the risk of having a stroke and of developing kidney disease, and can cause problems for other organs in the body. If a person has high blood pressure for a long period of time (*emphasise the long period of time*), and it has not been treated, then their heart muscle can become enlarged to compensate for the extra pressure. This can sometimes result in the heart not pumping as efficiently as it should. This condition is called *heart failure*. It is therefore important that we manage blood pressure effectively to reduce the risk of these problems developing or to help manage them well in the longer term. It might be that before your cardiac event you were diagnosed with high blood pressure and were put on medication to help to lower it. It is also possible that some people had high blood pressure before their cardiac event but were unaware of it as they had not had their blood pressure checked for a long time.

> **Question to group: "When you last had your blood pressure recorded do you remember what the figures were?"**
> *Write the figures on the whiteboard. Ask the staff for their figures and write down one set of figures that is at the lower end (e.g. 100/60) so that low blood pressure can be explained later. Also mention that generally not many people are aware of what their blood pressure figures are. Explain that we would like everyone to "know their figures" in the future and to have the confidence to ask medical/nursing staff for them.*

Everybody's blood pressure is different and your blood pressure will change throughout the day depending on what you are doing. For instance, blood pressure will rise when you are exercising and will come down again when you stop. If you are feeling particularly anxious or stressed, your blood pressure will rise. If you relax, your blood pressure will come back down. These are normal responses. The problems with high blood pressure arise when the blood pressure stays high all of the time. Having one or two high readings does not necessarily mean that you have high blood pressure.

Blood pressure is measured by two figures. The top figure is called the systolic blood pressure and measures the pressure in your arteries when your heart is beating. The bottom figure is called the diastolic blood pressure and measures the pressure in the arteries when the heart is at rest between each beat. Blood pressure is measured in millimetres of mercury (mm/Hg).

What Should Your Blood Pressure Be?

> **Question to group: "Looking at the blood pressure figures on the board, do you think that any of the figures are too high or too low?"**

Having been diagnosed with coronary heart disease you now have a target for your blood pressure in order to reduce your risk of further problems.

> **Question to group: "Do you know what the target level is for your blood pressure following a cardiac event?"**

The target level is to aim for your blood pressure to be less than **130/80 mm/Hg** (at rest) as this will greatly reduce the risk of having another cardiac event and the development of other problems. Remember when you exercise or when you feel stressed it is normal for your blood pressure to rise. What we are looking for are the figures when you are at rest and feeling fairly relaxed.

Write the blood pressure target on the whiteboard. The whiteboard at this point may be as in Figure 7.7.

For most people there are no symptoms of high blood pressure, and you will only know what your blood pressure is if you have it measured, preferably at the doctor's surgery. We should not be unduly concerned about low blood pressure unless it causes us to feel dizzy or light-headed. Unlike high blood pressure, it is not adversely associated with other health conditions. If you are told that you have lower figures and you are feeling well, then it is not something you should be unduly worried about.

How can we Lower our Blood Pressure?

> **Question to group: "How can we lower our blood pressure?"**
> *Ask the group to contribute and list the correct answers (these are in Figure 7.8) in bullet points on the board. Go back and explain each answer in more detail when you have a full list.*

This is linked to:

- Coronary heart disease
- Stroke
- Heart failure
- Kidney problems

What do the figures mean?

Examples:

160/85   110/60   180/90   100/60   mmHG

What is the target blood pressure for people with coronary heart disease?

Target: less than 130/80 mmHg

Know Your Figures!

Figure 7.7 High blood pressure

- Medication
- Relaxation
- Stop smoking
- Alcohol in moderation
- Weight management
- Regular exercise
- Reducing salt
- Eating a healthy diet

Figure 7.8 How can you achieve the target blood pressure of 130/80 mmHg?

Medication is one way of reducing our blood pressure. All of you will be on medication to reduce the risk of having a further cardiac event, and some of these medications can help to reduce your blood pressure. We will talk more about medication in Week 7 of the programme. For people who have had high blood pressure for some time it is common to be on two or more medications to help lower the blood pressure.

Relaxation is an important skill to learn as it can help to lower blood pressure. This can be useful in the general management of high blood pressure, and even more so at times of stress.

Stopping smoking can help to reduce our blood pressure.

Drinking alcohol in moderation can also help to control our blood pressure.

Weight management will help to control blood pressure, as being over-weight will increase the risk of a raised blood pressure. Losing weight will help to lower our blood pressure.

Regular exercise can lower both the systolic and diastolic blood pressure by up to 10 mm/Hg.

Reducing salt in the diet can also help to lower blood pressure. We will talk more about salt in Week 5 of the programme, when we discuss diet and coronary heart disease.

Eating a healthy diet. Again we will discuss this in Week 5 of the programme.

If you are looking at the list above and thinking that you need to make several changes to your lifestyle in order to help lower your blood pressure then it is advisable to prioritise these changes and make them one at a time in order to increase the prospect of maintaining them for life. We will discuss this in more detail next week!

Blood pressure target and lifestyle information in this chapter has been adapted from British Cardiac Society et al. (2005) and Williams et al. (2004).

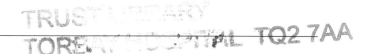
Chapter 8

Activities to Avoid, Making Changes for Life and Cholesterol (Week 4)

Session Plan for Week 4

1. Activities to Avoid at the Moment (10 minutes)
2. Exercise Practical (45 minutes)
   Tea and coffee break (15 minutes)
3. Mind and Body Relaxation (5 minutes)
4. Making Changes for Life (30 minutes)
5. Cholesterol (15 minutes)

---

1. Activities to Avoid at the Moment

Aim of the talk: to introduce patients to the idea that a thorough warm-up and cool-down is important in allowing safe and effective exercise.

It is a good idea at this point to check the group's understanding of the main messages concerning exercise covered in the previous weeks of the programme (i.e. frequency, intensity, time and type).

Question to group: "What type of exercise do you think would *not* be advisable in the early stages of your recovery from a cardiac event?"

Typical responses given are:

- *Heavy lifting*
- *Digging*
- *Pushing/pulling*

These responses can be written on the board as in Figure 8.1.

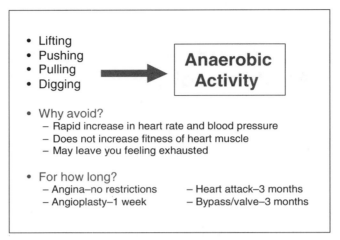

Figure 8.1 Activities to avoid

Activities such as heavy lifting or pushing and pulling (furniture for example) are typical **anaerobic** activities. Anaerobic exercise does not use oxygen as a fuel. The reason for this is that when, for example, we lift something that is heavy there is no time for our working muscles to be supplied the extra oxygen that they need to perform the task. These kinds of activity tend to be high-intensity and carried out over a short period of time. They tend to be short, sharp bursts of activity rather than gradual and prolonged (as in aerobic exercise). In the early stages of recovery from a cardiac event it is not ideal to be doing anaerobic exercise.

Question to group: "How long should we avoid doing anaerobic activities after a cardiac event?"

The period of time that you should avoid doing anaerobic activities after a cardiac event varies depending on what type of cardiac event you have experienced.

For patients who have experienced angina there are no restrictions. For patients who have experienced angioplasty it is one week. For patients who have experienced a heart attack or valve/bypass surgery the advice is three months. When this time has passed it is very important to build these activities back into your life gradually using the pacing principles discussed in Week 1 of the programme. For example, if you have not done any form of lifting activity for some time you will have lost some muscular strength.

What Would We Regard as Heavy Lifting?

What is regarded as heavy lifting will vary from individual to individual. A 90-year-old woman may find a certain item, such as a chair, extremely heavy to lift, whereas a 50-year-old man may find it relatively light. A good rule of thumb is that heavy lifting will be anything that makes us tense up our shoulders and forces us to hold our breath as we attempt to lift it.

The exception to this is following a coronary artery bypass graft, when we should not be lifting anything more than 10 pounds in weight within the first three months of the operation. This roughly equates to a kettle full of water.

2. Exercise Practical

Following the talk a practical exercise session is held using a circuit format to allow individuals of different abilities to work together.

Break for tea and coffee.

3. Mind and Body Relaxation

First of all ask how the group are progressing with the abdominal breathing that they were taught in Week 2 of the programme. Re-emphasise that abdominal breathing is a simple but powerful form of relaxation that can be used almost anywhere and at any time. Like any skill, it needs to be practised in order to improve and to gain the most benefit from it. Ask about the red dots and whether they have acted as a useful reminder for the group to take a couple of the abdominal breaths. Most groups find them very useful! Hand out a relaxation CD to each member of the group.

The first part of this session is going to focus on using the relaxation CD that we have given you. We will then talk about making changes for life, and finally the cardiac nurse will talk about cholesterol and why it is important in relation to coronary heart disease. We introduce the subject of cholesterol this week because next week we will be talking about diet and coronary heart disease, and we will want to discuss some of the other factors in our diet that are important in relation to CHD. Cholesterol is an important factor with regard to our diet, but it is not the only one, so we will attempt to put it into context in this session.

> **Question to group: "Why do we need to relax?"**

We talked in Week 2 about how relaxation is important in helping us to deal with stress and to cope with the stressful situations that we may face. We also mentioned that relaxation can help to lower our blood pressure, improve our sleep and our mood and reduce tension. However, relaxation is a skill and it takes time to become good at relaxing.

When we are relaxed the adrenaline level in our blood goes down, and this makes us feel calm. As we mentioned in Week 2 when we talked about stress, adrenaline is the key element in the "stress response" that puts up our heart rate, blood pressure and breathing rate, making us feel tense. To reduce this adrenaline response we need to learn ways of using relaxation effectively. The CD that we have given you can help you to relax better, but, like the abdominal breathing, the relaxation techniques on the CD need to be learnt and practised if you are to benefit from them.

Before you start we suggest that you:

- Give yourself half an hour to listen to the whole CD
- Find somewhere quiet and warm
- Make sure that you will not be interrupted
- Sit or lie down comfortably

If your mind wanders while you are listening to the CD try not to worry or get annoyed, just start listening again and carry on. As we mentioned previously, relaxation takes time. At first it may not seem easy or natural but if you practise then it will become increasingly easier over time.

There are three relaxation techniques on the CD. The first is deep muscle relaxation.

Deep Muscle Relaxation

On the CD, deep muscle relaxation comprises a series of exercises which covers all of the major muscle groups in the body, alternately tensing and relaxing. The easiest way to relax muscles is to tense them first and then to relax them. We can hold tension in our muscles without even realising it, and it can become a "normal" state for us. For instance we may hold tension in our face (*tense forehead into frown*) or in our shoulders (*hunch up shoulders*) or in our hands (*clench fists*). However, if we are aware that we are gradually becoming more tense then we have already taken the first step towards doing something about it.

Deep muscle relaxation is a very effective way of increasing our awareness of the tension that we hold in our body. Over time many people lose a sense of the difference between tension and relaxation. Deep muscle relaxation can help us to regain that understanding, helping us to identify the difference between feeling tense and feeling relaxed.

Ideally we need to do this exercise routine at least once a day for two or three weeks to begin to build up our skills. Once we have identified which particular muscle groups tend to tense us, we can focus on these areas during the day.

Question to group: "Why is tension bad for us?"

Muscles which are tense are working hard, so being tense can make us exhausted, even if we have been sitting in a chair all day. Muscle tension can also cause peculiar aches and pains, headaches, a stiff neck, and unusual chest sensations, as well as raising our blood pressure. Learning to reduce our muscle tension can help with all of these symptoms.

The second relaxation technique on the CD is called mental relaxation.

Mental Relaxation

Remember: the mind and body work together. Sometimes we can carry an awful lot of strain around in our minds. Consequently, mental relaxation is important; if you try to relax physically and your mind is not relaxing as well, then worries, or even everyday thoughts, will work against any relaxation. Use your imagination in a form of mental relaxation.

Some Tips for Successful Mental Relaxation

Make yourself comfortable: When you are physically comfortable, it can help to imagine an experience or a place that has in the past made you feel relaxed and happy. It might be:

- Your favourite place in the countryside
- A holiday lying on the beach in the sun
- Sitting by a stream or river listening to the sound of the water
- A comfortable chair looking out on a favourite view
- Being outside on a warm evening watching the stars appear
- Sitting in front of an open log fire

Recall memories from all your senses: Look at the colours. Experience the feeling on your face and body. Feel the warmth or the breeze. Notice the sounds and the smells. Counting down slowly from say 300 may make you feel more relaxed.

Don't worry if you have difficulty with this approach. Often when we are feeling stressed it is hard to concentrate. As our stress levels come down, we can sometimes find these exercises easier to follow.

The last of the relaxation techniques on the CD is called autogenic relaxation.

Autogenic Relaxation

Autogenic means self-generated, and autogenic relaxation involves an interaction between our mind and our body, using our thoughts to create a physical response. It is the most advanced technique on the CD and can therefore take a bit longer to perfect.

With deep muscle relaxation the focus is on the physical effect on our body. With mental relaxation the focus is on thinking and our mental processes. With autogenic relaxation the two are in combination.

We know from research that we can influence our circulation simply by concentrating on it. If we concentrate on making one hand feel warmer than the other, with a bit of practice we can actually change the temperature of that hand or indeed other parts of the body. We know that hand temperature is linked to stress levels because when we are stressed our blood supply is directed towards our major organs as part of the stress response. This means that our hands and feet receive less circulation and are likely to feel colder.

Autogenic relaxation increases the circulation to our extremities such as our hands, feet, ears and nose. By imagining feelings of warmth and heaviness in different parts of the body we can create real physical changes as we relax. It takes practice but many people find it easy to master, providing another means of relaxing and maintaining relaxation. Research has also shown that practising this form of relaxation can lessen perceived angina symptoms.

Tips for using the relaxation CD

1. The CD is first and foremost a learning aid. It is not designed to just make us relaxed while listening to it.
2. Falling asleep while listening to the CD is common but not particularly helpful as we will not then learn the relaxation techniques (however, for some people who are having problems sleeping the CD can be used in bed to help them get to sleep).
3. While listening to the CD your aim is to be "relaxed but alert" so that you are aware of the sensation of feeling relaxed.

(Continued)

---

4. Continue to use the abdominal breathing during the day. Do not just rely on a "quick fix" of relaxation at the end of the day by using the CD. The CD becomes ineffective very quickly if you do this.

5. Set aside a regular time each day to listen to the CD in order to build up relaxation skills.

4. Making Changes for Life

The aim of this part of the session is to help you to make changes to your lifestyle (if you decide that there are changes that you want to make) and to maintain those changes for life. We will look at why it can be important for some people to make changes after a cardiac event, how to go about making those changes and finally how to maintain the changes in the long term.

Why Make Changes for Life?

In Week 1 when we discussed the risk factors for coronary heart disease we discovered that, although there is not a cure, it is a condition that can be managed very well. We also discovered that there are two sides to the management of coronary heart disease. First, there is the medical management, through the various interventions that we discussed in Week 1 (such as coronary artery bypass grafting, angioplasty and stents) and through prescribed medication. Second, there is the management of the risk factors for coronary heart disease through lifestyle modification. Coronary heart disease can be managed very well through medication and lifestyle changes, but importantly the benefits of any changes that are made will only last for as long as those changes are maintained. There is good evidence that positive lifestyle changes to the risk factors for coronary heart disease, such as stopping smoking, increasing exercise, reducing excessive alcohol consumption and changing diet, can (along with taking cardiac medication) help to halt any further build-up of fatty plaques in the coronary arteries and reduce the incidence of further cardiac events. The benefits are only evident, however, while these lifestyle changes are maintained. If we maintain lifestyle change life-long, the risk of further problems is reduced life-long. If not, then a greater risk of a further cardiac event returns.

> **Question to group: "Has anybody made any lifestyle changes since their cardiac event that they would like to tell us about?"**
> *Wait for responses and acknowledge these changes, or any problems with making changes that individuals may have had.*

Making changes can be difficult for all of us, as often the behaviours that we are trying to change, such as in our diet, smoking or alcohol consumption, can be behaviours that we have been doing for many years, sometimes even decades. In some cases the behaviours have been passed down through our family. It can therefore be extremely difficult to change a behaviour that you have practised for 40 or 50 years. However, if we go about making lifestyle changes in an appropriate way, it is possible to make successful changes to long-standing behaviours and to maintain these changes for life.

An important aspect of behaviour change is that you must *want* to make the change in the first place. If you are making changes because you feel pressure from others, but don't believe personally that it is a change that you should be making, then there is very little chance that you will maintain the change for life. Some of the group may feel that there are no changes that they need to make to their lifestyle. Others may be thinking that it is not the right time for them to, for instance, give up smoking, but that they do want to give up at some stage. That is fine. Some will be ready to make changes now, while others have already done so and will be looking to keep those changes going. The important thing is that if you *intend* to make a change then it is likely that you will, at some stage, end up making that change even if it is not immediately.

Making Changes

If you are making a change to your lifestyle, there are four steps that will make the process easier. (The exception to this is if you are trying to stop smoking. Smoking is a complex behaviour that involves physical and psychological addiction and some people will require specialist help to be successful in stopping. This specialist help is available through trained smoking cessation advisers to whom a referral can be made if necessary. Please talk to a member of the team who will be able to help.)

Decide What You Want to Change *(Write This on the Whiteboard)*

The first step towards making a change for life is to decide what it is that you want to change. This could be reducing your alcohol consumption, increasing exercise or eating more fruit and vegetables. Making a decision to go ahead and make the change is also very important. We often have a vague idea that we would like to cut down on our drinking or eat more fruit and vegetables, but we end up never getting round to it. Deciding to make the change and having the intention to follow it through is very important in being successful with a behaviour change.

Prioritise the Changes *(Write This on the Whiteboard)*

Prioritising the changes that you are going to make is important for two reasons. First, if you have more than one change that you intend to make then it is important to make those changes one at a time. Sometimes we can try and change too many things at once and end up losing focus on what we are trying to achieve, or feeling overwhelmed by it all. This can result in us quickly returning to our old ways. As we mentioned earlier, we need changes to be life-long, not just for a few months. Second, it is important to prioritise changes in order to build confidence and ultimately to be more successful in maintaining the changes. For example, it might be that the easier change for an individual to make might be to do an extra session of exercise a week rather than attempting to reduce their alcohol consumption (which they perceive as being more difficult to achieve). The confidence gained by that person in successfully managing to increase the amount that they are exercising may then help when tackling the more difficult issue for them of a reduction in alcohol consumption. Other people will attempt the most difficult behavioural change first with the view that if they can achieve that change then they will be confident that they can master any others. It will be different for different people, but the important thing is that we don't try and do it all at once!

Set Achievable Goals and Pace *(Write This on the Whiteboard)*

When we make changes it is crucial that the goals that we set ourselves are achievable and that we are sensible in the way that we go about achieving those goals. We can return to the goal-setting ladder that we talked about in Week 1 (*draw goal-setting ladder on the whiteboard*). It might be, for example, that we have decided that our priority is to eat more fruit and vegetables. Currently let's say that we do not eat any fruit and vegetables (*this is our baseline – write "0" on the bottom rung of the ladder*). In setting our goal we have decided to eat 15 portions of fruit and vegetables a day, starting tomorrow, and we are hoping to keep this change going life-long (*write "15" at the top of the ladder next to "Goal"*).

> ## Question to group:"Does this sound like an achievable goal?"

Certainly if our baseline was that we were currently not eating any fruit and vegetables and we decided to start eating 15 portions a day then the chances of keeping this going for a few days, let alone life-long, would be virtually nil! A more sensible approach would be to set an achievable specific goal, such as eating five portions of fruit and vegetables a day, and then pacing ourselves up the goal-setting ladder to achieve that goal (*change the "15" to "5" at the top of the ladder*). If we were not eating any fruit and vegetables at all, then starting with one portion a day would be the most sensible approach until it became a habit for us. We could then move on to a second portion, and so on. When attempting to make new habits it can help to be practising the new behaviours at the same time each day so that we develop a routine. For instance, putting dried fruit on cereal every day at breakfast time can quickly become a habit. Although it may seem unusual at first, after a few weeks it can seem unusual to have cereal without it! It is then time to move up a rung on the ladder and consider fitting in a second portion (*show this on the ladder*). Eventually over time (and it may take some months) we will achieve the goal that we have set ourselves. By pacing our changes (and most, although not all, changes that we make can be paced successfully) we are much more likely to keep the changes going long-term.

Keep a Diary *(Write This on the Whiteboard)*

It is important to know as much as we can about the behaviours that we are trying to change as it can be difficult to reduce, increase or give up some of these behaviours. Writing down details of our behaviours—whether they are to do with drinking, eating or exercising—allows us to understand in detail different aspects of them, and our thoughts and feelings about those behaviours, and how we might do things differently. Particularly important are details about:

- Antecedents—what happens before the behaviour, or the "trigger" for the behaviour
- Behaviours—what we want to change—e.g. eating less fatty food or doing more exercise
- Consequences—the consequences of the behaviour; this can relate to how we think or feel

If we take eating fatty food as an example, there are often a number of antecedents or triggers that lead us to eat certain foods that are not so good for

Example	Antecedent	Behaviour	Consequences
Eating	Feeling fed up	Eat some biscuits	Feel more cheerful
Alternative	*Feeling fed up*	*Go for a walk; talk to friend or partner*	*Feel more cheerful*

Figure 8.2 Diary of changing eating habits

us, such as feeling stressed, getting home from work, or having a midday cup of coffee. The example here (*write on the whiteboard as in Figure 8.2*) shows what a diary entry might look like if we were planning to change an eating habit. The diary entry can help in trying to understand the behaviour that we want to change in detail and focuses on alternative behaviours that can help in breaking a particular habit.

In this example a behavioural substitution can be effective in helping to change our eating habits. Going for a walk or talking to a friend or our partner can have the same consequence as the behaviour that we are trying to change. In fact the behaviour that we are trying to change, whether that is eating unhealthy food, drinking alcohol or smoking, tends to only help us to cope with some of our negative thoughts and feelings in the short term. It may seem to have an immediate positive benefit to us (such as helping us to relax or improve our mood) but in the long term it can be a harmful risk factor for coronary heart disease, as we discovered in Week 1. Often the behaviours that we substitute for it—such as regular exercise or talking things through—can prove to be much more effective long-term coping strategies.

FIT

When we consider how to change our behaviours, for most of them we can focus on one of the following: the **frequency** of the behaviour, the **intensity** of the behaviour, or the **time** that the behaviour takes (*write Frequency, Intensity and Time on the whiteboard as in Figure 8.3*).

For example, if we decided to cut down on our alcohol consumption (and this was our priority) then we could look at changing either the frequency, the intensity or the time that we spent engaging in this behaviour.

It is important to remember to change just one of these elements and not to try and change all of them at once. It is also important to remember the pacing

	Before	**After**
Frequency	Go to the pub 4 times/week	Go to the pub 3 times/week
Intensity	Drink pints of beer	Drink pints of shandy Drink half-pints of beer
Time	Go out at 8.00pm	Go out at 9.00pm

Figure 8.3 Reducing alcohol consumption

ladder that we referred to earlier when setting our goals so that we reduce our consumption gradually. For example, it is possible that if we had been going to the pub four times a week and changed immediately to going just once a week it could potentially seem like too much of a change. Our social life might be badly affected and we could end up giving up and returning to the pub four times a week.

If we are to make lasting changes it is important to remember to pace ourselves properly.

Frequency	If we usually went to the pub four times a week then we could initially reduce this to three times a week, with the aim of reducing it further if this was necessary.
Intensity	We could still go to the pub four times a week, but rather than drink pints of beer we could drink pints of shandy or half-pints of beer. Alternatively we could have a soft drink if we were drinking in rounds. Again it is important to remember the pacing ladder and to reduce the intensity gradually.
Time	We could still go to the pub four times a week and still drink pints of beer but we could go later in the evening. By spending less time at the pub we can reduce the amount of alcohol that we drink. This only works as long as we do not increase the speed of our drinking while we are at the pub!

As mentioned earlier, making changes to our lifestyle is not necessarily an easy process, and some changes can be difficult to maintain in the long term. Being aware of this and recognising that **setbacks** can occur is an important part of successfully making and maintaining behaviour changes.

Setbacks and Maintaining Behaviour Change

Most changes that we make don't go *exactly* as we planned. Setbacks are a normal part of life, and it is no different when we make changes and try to maintain them. However, if we recognise that setbacks can occur, and consider in advance how we might cope with them, then we are more likely to keep our changes going rather than reverting to our original behaviours. Some ways of coping with potential setbacks are to:

Avoid Complacency

One of the most common reasons for returning to a behaviour that we have tried to change (smoking is a common example) is that we become complacent. We sometimes think that by "just having the odd one" we will be all right, but rapidly find that we have returned to our previous behaviour. If you do find yourself in this situation then try and view it as a minor hiccup, and remain determined not to restart. Having one cigarette at a time of intense stress, for example, doesn't mean that you are back to being a "twenty a day" person! Consider how well you have done in not smoking, or drinking alcohol, or eating unhealthy food for the past few weeks or months (or even years), and then put it down as a minor setback and continue onwards.

Be Assertive

If you are offered a cigarette, or cake, or extra drink that you do not want, then a simple, "No thank you" works better than "I'd love to really but I'm trying to stop/cut down". Sometimes other people will see this kind of response as the green light to push you further. As mentioned previously, it can be beneficial if you can avoid situations where you think this might occur, especially in the early stages of making a change.

Coping With Craving

Be prepared to cope with the occasional strong urge to smoke or eat certain foods. These urges do not tend to last long, but being aware that you may have them and that they will pass is an important part of maintaining changes.

Reward Yourself

Plan rewards for successfully making a change and reward yourself from the start. It might be a meal out or going to a show or the cinema. We all need positive and enjoyable things to look forward to, so planning them in as an incentive to keep your lifestyle change going is a sensible step towards maintaining that change for life.

The cardiac nurse will now talk about cholesterol for the remainder of this session.

5. Cholesterol

In the final part of the session we are going to talk about cholesterol. We will discuss what cholesterol is and what cholesterol is required for in our bodies. We will then discuss where it comes from and the part that it plays in coronary heart disease. Following a cardiac event there is a target set for your cholesterol level, and we will discuss how we can lower our cholesterol levels in order to try and reach this target.

What is Cholesterol?

Cholesterol is one of the lipids or fatty substances which is carried in the bloodstream. We need cholesterol as it is an essential part of the make-up of our cell membranes; it is used in the production of some hormones and also in the production of bile salts.

Question to group: "Where does cholesterol come from?"

Most of the cholesterol in our bodies is produced by our liver, and the rest comes from our diet. The amount that we produce is affected by what we eat, in particular food that is high in saturated fat. It is also affected by certain lifestyle factors (which we will discuss later), and by hereditary factors.

Question to group: "Why are we concerned with your cholesterol level now that you have coronary heart disease?"

We know that we need a certain amount of cholesterol for the reasons we discussed earlier. The problem arises when we have too much of it. We know that if we have too much cholesterol in our system it can be laid down in the walls of the coronary arteries, causing further narrowing.

What Should Our Cholesterol Level Be?

> **Question to group: "Do you know what your cholesterol level is?"**
> *Consider writing these levels on the whiteboard, then go on to explain that these are figures for "total" cholesterol.*

Cholesterol levels vary from individual to individual. The national average for the UK is around 5.7–5.8, and these figures represent our *total cholesterol level*. The cholesterol that we produce needs to be transported around the body in the blood to the cells which need it. It travels in the blood by attaching itself to a protein and thus becomes a "lipoprotein". There are two main types of lipoprotein: high-density lipoprotein (HDL) and low-density lipoprotein (LDL).

LDL cholesterol is often called the "bad cholesterol" as, if we have too much of it, it can be dumped inside the walls of the coronary arteries. HDL cholesterol is sometimes known as the "good cholesterol", as it scavenges for any excess cholesterol and carries it back to the liver where it is processed. It is therefore important for us to aim to have higher levels of HDL and lower levels of LDL.

There are now national targets for total cholesterol and LDL cholesterol for people with coronary heart disease.

> **Question to group: "How low should your total cholesterol level be if you have coronary heart disease?"**

Cholesterol is measured in millimoles per litre (mmol/l) and for people with coronary heart disease the target for cholesterol is (*write these figures on the whiteboard*):

- total cholesterol level to be: lower than 4.0 mmol/l
- LDL cholesterol to be: lower than 2.0 mmol/l

For people who have had a cardiac event: if your cholesterol level was below these figures before your cardiac event then we would still want a reduction of 25 per cent in your total cholesterol level and a 30 per cent reduction in your LDL cholesterol. This is because we know that the lower your cholesterol level is, the less likely you are to have a further cardiac event. Following a cardiac event your GP surgery will monitor your cholesterol (with the aim of meeting these targets) through a simple blood test. It is therefore important for you to know what your cholesterol levels are (both total cholesterol level and LDL level) to make sure that you are meeting the national targets.

How to Lower and Improve Our Cholesterol Levels

Question to group: "How can we lower our cholesterol levels to meet the national targets?"
Write the correct answers on the whiteboard in bullet points and then explain in more detail (see Figure 8.4.)

The main way that we can reduce our total cholesterol level following a cardiac event is through **medication**. Everybody who has coronary heart disease should be on medication to lower their total cholesterol level, the most common of which are called **statins**. Statins work on the liver to reduce the amount of cholesterol that is produced and lower both the total cholesterol level and also the LDL level. It is important to keep taking the statins long-term; if you stop taking them your cholesterol will return to its previous level.

Reducing saturated fat in our diet is the second way in which we can influence our cholesterol levels. Saturated fats are found in dairy foods, in the fat on meat and in processed foods. We will talk about saturated fats in more detail in Week 5. Saturated fats raise both the total cholesterol level and LDL cholesterol level.

It should also be noted that eating **oily fish** can help to lower triglycerides, another lipid, as well as being protective of the heart in other ways which we

- **Total cholesterol level to be: lower than 4 mmol/l**
- **LDL cholesterol to be: lower than 2.0 mmol/l**
  How can you achieve these targets?
  - *Medication*
  - *Reducing saturated fat in diet*
  - *Regular exercise*
  - *Weight management*
  - *Stop smoking*
  - *Alcohol in moderation*

Figure 8.4 Targets for cholesterol if you have coronary heart disease

will discuss in Week 5. Replacing some of the saturated fats in the diet with monounsaturated fats (i.e. olive oil, rapeseed oil) can also be beneficial, as these can lower LDL cholesterol levels without lowering the HDL cholesterol levels.

Regular exercise can help to boost the level of HDL, which in turn reduces the amount of cholesterol that is dumped in our coronary arteries.

Being overweight also influences our cholesterol levels. Losing weight will help to lower cholesterol levels.

Stopping smoking reduces the damaging effects on the artery walls that can subsequently lead to a build-up of cholesterol.

Alcohol in moderation can boost the HDL cholesterol and therefore have a protective effect. Alcohol in excess can have a damaging effect on the heart muscle as well as raising triglycerides, which is a "bad" lipid. If you do not drink alcohol at present, however, we would not recommend that you start!

In summary:

Cholesterol is a fatty substance carried in the bloodstream and is needed for cell production and hormone development. However, if we have too much it can be laid down in the walls of the coronary arteries, causing them to become narrowed. Now that we know you have coronary heart disease it is important to aim to get your total cholesterol and LDL cholesterol levels as low as possible, and raise the level of HDL cholesterol. With medication and lifestyle changes most people will be able to meet these targets. **From now on we would encourage you to ask for your cholesterol results to ensure that you know that you are at the recommended targets**.

A small number of people may need further advice from a lipidologist (a specialist who is an expert in lipids) to try to achieve these targets. These are usually people who have cholesterol levels much higher than the national average; this is often caused by a genetic condition.

Target and lifestyle information for cholesterol in this chapter is adapted from British Cardiac Society et al. (2005) and British Heart Foundation (2007b).

Chapter 9

Enough or Too Much Exercise? Diet and Coronary Heart Disease (Week 5)

Session Plan for Week 5

1. Enough or Too Much Exercise? (10 minutes)
2. Exercise Practical (45 minutes)
    Tea and coffee break (15 minutes)
3. Diet and Coronary Heart Disease (50 minutes)

1. Enough or too Much Exercise?

Aim of the talk: to reinforce the pacing message and get individuals to recognise the common signs and symptoms of overdoing exercise.

At this stage patients will have been exercising on the programme for three weeks and may have been completing their own exercise programmes at home. They will all have experienced occasions when they have misjudged the amount of exercise that they could comfortably complete and they may have been unsure of how to manage this type of situation.

In this session it is useful to get patients and partners to talk about how they would recognise if they were overdoing it during an exercise session. Most individuals will be able to report an experience of when they have overdone their exercise (in the last few weeks) and how they felt as a result. This session can be started by asking the group once more about the frequency, intensity, time and type of exercise that they should ideally be doing and listing the responses on the whiteboard.

Question to group: "How do we know if we are overdoing our exercise (doing too much)?"

This question can be divided into two parts: (1) during exercise and (2) following exercise (i.e. later/the next day). The responses can be written on the whiteboard as in Figure 9.1 below.

- **Enough**
  - Aerobic exercise
  - 3–5 times a week
  - 60–75% of maximum heart rate/somewhat hard
- **Too much**
  - Ways of recognising if you are overdoing things

During exercise
Breathless–unable to say phone number
Heart rate above training range
Dizzy/light-headed
Muscle aches and pains
Get angina
Feel exhausted
Poor co-ordination
Have to stop exercise and rest

Following exercise (later/ the next day)
Feel exhausted
Muscles aches and pains
Have to rest–no exercise possible

Figure 9.1 Exercise: not enough . . . too much?

When we are building up an exercise programme it can require some trial and error. When increasing our exercise it is important to build it up in small increments and then reflect on this increase and how it felt before increasing the exercise any further. This is where our exercise diaries are invaluable, as they give a very detailed picture of our exercise regime. It can be very useful to look back at the previous day to determine possible causes of tiredness or exhaustion.

So, for example, if someone was to increase their daily walking time from 20 to 30 minutes it might be quite a big jump for them (and subsequently they may find it too much of an increase). This could leave them feeling tired and achy. This individual would potentially then need to reassess things and maybe reduce their exercise to, for example, 25 minutes. Once they feel that they can cope with that amount of walking they could then increase it to 30 minutes and assess once more.

It is also important to make patients and partners aware of the effect of other daily activities (i.e. housework, shopping, visiting friends, hospital visits) on their recovery. All of these types of activity should be taken into consideration when planning an exercise regime. For example, it may be that the 30-minute walk is an appropriate amount of exercise for an individual, but coupled with a busy day of shopping and visiting friends that person is left feeling overtired the next day.

It can be a complex task trying to plan and pace daily activities after a cardiac event, but it is vitally important in order to achieve the best possible recovery. Overdoing things won't do any damage to your heart, but it may set you back in terms of your recovery.

2. Exercise Practical

Following the talk a practical exercise session is held using a circuit format to allow individuals of different abilities to work together.
Break for tea and coffee

3. Diet and Coronary Heart Disease

In this session we are going to talk about diet and coronary heart disease. In particular we are going to talk about the most recent evidence and advice that we have for healthy eating following a cardiac event which can help to reduce the risk of having another cardiac event, as well as influencing some of the risk factors we discussed in Week 1.

In the last session we talked about cholesterol, the part it plays in relation to coronary heart disease and what we can do to lower our cholesterol levels, and diet plays an important part in this. Diabetes is a risk factor for coronary heart disease, and diet is an important part of the management of this condition. Other risk factors which can be influenced by diet will be high blood pressure and being overweight. We will mention cholesterol today, but there are five other main aspects of your diet that we want to focus on.

For anyone who has diabetes the following recommendations should go alongside your diet for diabetes. If anyone feels they need an update on the diabetic diet there should be support at your GP practice. If this is not available then please let us know and we can refer you to one of the dieticians within cardiac rehabilitation.

Another risk factor you may need support with is weight management. If this is your goal, check at your GP surgery to see if they have a practice nurse who can advise on controlling your weight. If a nurse is not available, again we can refer you to one of our dieticians. There is further information in your handbook.

> **Question to group: "What do you think are the five most important factors concerning your diet following a cardiac event?"**
>
> *Wait for replies from the group and write the correct answers on the whiteboard.*

The five areas of our diet that we are going to focus on today are:

- Oily fish
- Fats
- Fruit and vegetables
- Salt
- Alcohol

We will now discuss each of these in more detail. You will be advised to eat more of some of these items and less of others. The advice given is based on the basic principles of the "Mediterranean diet", which research has shown to be cardio-protective.

Oily Fish

Question to group: "Which fish are the oily fish?"

Wait for responses and write: herring, salmon, sardines, trout, pilchards, kippers, mackerel, fresh tuna (though not tinned as it does not contain high enough levels of omega-3) and halibut (a white fish that contains high levels of omega-3) on the whiteboard.

Oily fish is at the top of the list in terms of the important things we should be adding to our diet following a cardiac event. This is because oily fish have a special substance called omega-3 oil that is contained in the flesh of the fish and which is beneficial to our hearts. Studies have shown that eating oily fish regularly following a cardiac event can significantly reduce the risk of a further cardiac event. Oily fish also has a stabilising effect on the heart and makes blood less likely to clot. White fish (such as cod, plaice, haddock, etc.) is a good food to have in our diet, but it does not contain the omega-3 fish oil in sufficient amounts to be beneficial. If you are not able to eat oily fish regularly then please discuss it with your GP, as he or she may now be in a position to prescribe a supplement for you. If you have had a recent heart attack (within the last three months), then we have a letter we can give you to take to your GP to support this request. If your GP is not happy to prescribe this, fish oil supplements can be bought from chemists, supermarkets and health food shops, and will help to protect your heart in the same way.

The omega-3 recommendations are as follows (*write these on the whiteboard*):

If you have *not* had a heart attack:

- Aim for one to two portions of fish a week (oily or white), 1 portion of which should be oily.
  Or
- An omega-3 fish oil supplement equal to 500 mg of "EPA + DHA" fish oils per day.

If you *have* had a heart attack within the last three months:

- Aim for two to four portions of oily fish a week (one portion = 140 g or 5 oz).
  Or:
- An omega-3 fish oil supplement equal to 1000 mg of "EPA + DHA" fish oils per day.

Research has demonstrated that the benefits to cardiac health are seen when these measures are initiated within three months of a cardiac event and maintained for up to four years.

If you eat oily fish regularly in the amounts recommended above, then you do not need to take the fish oil supplements as well. Studies have shown that there is no additional benefit to be gained from consuming more oily fish than the recommended amounts.

If you take cod liver oil for your joints this generally does not contain enough omega-3. You can switch to the omega-3 fish oil and this will give you benefits to your joints as well as protecting your heart.

After the discussion on oily fish the whiteboard may resemble Figure 9.2.

Fats

The second important factor to consider in our diet following a cardiac event is fats.

Question to group: "What are the different types of fat in our diet?"
Wait for responses and write "saturated fat", "trans fats", "monounsaturated fats" and "polyunsaturated fat" on the whiteboard.

There are four types of fat found in food. The type and the amount of fat in our diet can have an effect on coronary heart disease.

Fat is high in calories, and having too much can contribute to being overweight, which is, as we have mentioned, one of the risk factors for coronary heart disease. Also, the type of fat that we eat can influence our good and bad cholesterol levels.

Oily fish

Fats   Oily fish—reduces risk of further

Fruit and vegetables   cardiac event by 30%

Salt

Alcohol

Examples of oily fish

herring, salmon, sardines, fresh tuna, halibut

How much fish is recommended for people with coronary heart disease?

Following a heart attack: 2–4 5 oz portions/week

Or supplement 500–1000 mg EPA + DHA per day

Maintain for 4 years

For other cardiac events: 1–2 5 oz portions/week

Or supplement 500 mg EPA + DHA per day

Figure 9.2 Diet and coronary heart disease

Question to group: "In which foods do we find these fats?"
List examples of these foods under the headings on the whiteboard as in Table 9.1, *and then explain the effects on the good and bad cholesterol.*

Saturated Fats and Trans Fats

Eating foods high in saturated fats increases our cholesterol levels, particularly the "bad" LDL cholesterol. Trans fats are thought to have a similar effect. Therefore we should try to eat fewer saturated and trans fats.

Cutting the visible fat off meat, especially before cooking, can be a good start. Try to reduce frying and roasting and use more healthy cooking methods instead such as steaming, grilling and poaching. Eating processed foods less often will also help to reduce the amount of saturated fat (as well as the amount of salt) in our diet. Full-fat dairy foods can be high in saturated fat so using a low-fat version is one option. Alternatively if this is not to your taste then choosing a strong cheese, for instance, and grating instead of slicing it may mean that you use less. Cheeses lower in fat include cottage cheese, feta, mozzarella, edam and ricotta. We would not want to cut dairy foods out of our diet completely as they are an excellent source of calcium, but it may be that you decide that this is an area in which you can reduce either the *frequency* (the number of times that you eat cheese each week, for example) or the *intensity*

Table 9.1 Types and examples of fats and their effect on cholesterol

Saturated	Trans fats	Monounsaturated	Polyunsaturated
Butter	Pastry foods	Olive oil	Corn oil
Hard cheese	Cakes	Rapeseed oil	Sunflower oil
Processed meat foods	Biscuits	Some vegetable oils	Some nuts and seeds: walnuts,
Cakes	Hard margarines	Olive oil-based spread	Pine nuts, sesame seeds
Fatty meats	Any foods that	Avocado	Margarines
Some ready meals	are 'hydrogenated'	Some nuts and seeds: almonds,	
Lard	Cashews		
↑ LDL	↑ LDL	↓LDL protects HDL	↓ LDL ↓HDL

(e.g. using a lower-fat spread, or grating cheese so that you use less) of use, as we discussed in Week 4 on making changes for life.

Monounsaturated Fats

Monounsaturated fats in your diet can help to lower the level of "bad" cholesterol while maintaining the level of "good" cholesterol in your blood, and it therefore has a protective effect. We would advise that you replace some of the saturated fats in your diet with the monounsaturated fats as these are more beneficial. One example of this would be to swap from butter, which is highest in saturated fat, to an olive oil-based spread which is much lower in saturated fats and highest in monounsaturated fats.

Polyunsaturated Fat

Polyunsaturated fat is found most commonly in oily fish (omega-3 fish oils), sunflower oil, corn oil and soya oils. Having oily fish in the diet will give you enough polyunsaturated fats. There is no evidence that including more of these fats than this in your diet will be of any benefit.

Fruit and Vegetables

Write "Fruit and Vegetables" on the whiteboard.

> **Question to group: "What is the recommended daily intake for fruit and vegetables?"**

It is recommended that you should be eating at least *five portions a day* of fruit and vegetables, and that will give you a good variety of vitamins, minerals, antioxidants and soluble fibre. Eating a variety of fruit and vegetables with a variety of colours will give you: all the vitamins and minerals needed for good health; antioxidants, which are protective to our arteries; and fibre, which keeps us "regular" and also helps to lower cholesterol.

Question to group: "How many of you manage to eat five portions of fruit and vegetables a day?"

Some of you will be eating five a day but others may be finding this very difficult to achieve. We know that eating one portion of fruit and vegetables a day is better than eating none at all and that eating two portions is better than just the one, and so on. In terms of increasing the amount that you eat it is advisable to return to the **goal-setting ladder** that we talked about in Week 1, and to increase the number of portions one at a time. Once you have consolidated eating an extra portion each day (e.g. an apple mid-morning) and it has become habitual, then you can move on adding another portion. This will help to maintain the change in the longer term.

Question to group: "How much is a portion?"
Write correct answers on the whiteboard as in Figure 9.3.

When we talk about a *portion* of fruit and vegetables we are referring to around 80 grams, or 3 ounces, which translates as approximately a "handful". It is important to remember that each fruit or vegetable only counts once a day, so eating five apples will only count as one portion!

Tinned, frozen and dried fruit and vegetables all count towards the five a day, although a tablespoon of dried fruit will count as a portion.

An example of how you might incorporate five portions of fruit and vegetables into your day would be that you start the day with a glass of fruit juice, or alternatively have some chopped or dried fruit on a bowl of cereal. A piece of fruit as a mid-morning snack would take you up to two portions for the day and a bowl of salad or a small tin of beans on toast at lunchtime would make three. Two vegetables with dinner would make it up to five portions. Any more fruit and vegetables during the day would be a bonus! However, remember your pacing and that if you are only eating, for example, one portion a day don't jump straight to five a day, as you are unlikely to maintain the change life-long and your digestive system will not thank you for it either!

Aim for 5 portions a day

One portion = 80 g or 3oz = a handful

- **A medium apple, banana or orange**
- **Two medium-sized plums, satsumas or kiwi fruit**
- **A slice of melon**
- **Three heaped tablespoons of carrots, peas, etc.**
- **Two spears of broccoli/cauliflower**
- **A small tin of baked beans/chickpeas/kidney beans**
- **A bowl of vegetable soup**
- **A 150 ml glass of fruit juice**

Remember: a variety of colours!

Figure 9.3 Fruit and vegetables

Salt

Question to group: "Why is salt important with regard to coronary heart disease?"

Salt can have a detrimental effect on blood pressure, which is one of the *risk factors* for coronary heart disease. The recommended maximum intake for salt in the UK is 5–6 grams per day (which is approximately a teaspoonful). We tend to eat too much salt though, and the average daily salt intake is around 12 grams per day. Even if you do not have high blood pressure, reducing your salt intake can lead to beneficial effects on your blood pressure

Question to group: "How can we reduce the amount of salt in our diet?"
Write "Salt" on the whiteboard and then the suggestions from the group as in Figure 9.4.

The simplest way to cut down on the amount of salt that you eat is to add less when you are cooking or at the table. By cutting your salt intake down gradually over a period of a few weeks you may not notice a difference in taste. However, the majority of salt in our diet comes from processed foods. Foods such as bread, breakfast cereal, tinned soups, packet soups and sauces can all be

How can we reduce our intake of salt to a maximum of 6 g per day?

- Add less during cooking
- Try your food before adding salt at the table
- Use herbs and spices; vinegar, mustard, pepper, lemon juice instead of salt
- Eat fewer processed foods
- Try products which are unsalted or have less salt e.g. nuts and crisps
- Buy tinned fish/vegetables in water instead of brine

Check packet labels from time to time using the guide in the handbook

Figure 9.4 Salt contributes to high blood pressure

high in salt. It is worthwhile checking food labels to see the level of salt that is in a particular product. Some products are labelled telling us either the amount of salt or the amount of sodium in that product, which can be confusing. In your handbook there is a guide to help you to know how much is "a lot" and how much is "a little".

Salt replacement products such as LoSalt and So-Lo are low in sodium (which is the part of salt that affects blood pressure), but they are high in potassium, which can be harmful to your heart in large quantities. For this reason these products are not recommended.

Alcohol

There is some evidence to suggest that alcohol in moderation can be beneficial for coronary heart disease as it is associated with higher levels of "good" HDL cholesterol. The key word here is "moderation". Alcohol in larger amounts is associated with increased risk of coronary heart disease and other health problems. If you do not drink alcohol at present it is not suggested that you start.

Question to group: "What are the recommendations for alcohol intake if you have coronary heart disease?"
Write responses on white board as in Figure 9.5 and then go on to ask:
Question to group: "How much is a unit?"
Discuss further. A useful tool to give to patients if it is available is an "alcohol wheel" which works out the alcohol content in different volumes of alcohol, and the alcohol percentages of various drinks.

Men – max 3 units a day
no more than 21 units a week
Women – max 2 units a day
No more than 14 units a week

How much is a unit?

1 unit wine = small glass, 125 ml, 9% alcohol

1 unit beer/lager/cider = ½ pint ordinary strength, 3.5–5% alcohol

1 unit spirits = 25 ml

Single measure of aperitif

Remember: at least 2 alcohol-free days each week

Figure 9.5 Alcohol and coronary heart disease

It is also recommended that you have **at least** two alcohol-free days per week, and that you avoid binge-drinking, which would be having more than three units of alcohol over a one- to two-hour period.

It is important to remember that certain beers, lagers and ciders can be much stronger than others and will thus contain more units of alcohol. Home measures can also be much larger than pub measures. If you are looking to reduce your alcohol consumption but think it may be difficult, please speak to a member of the team or to your GP, who will be able to advise you further.

In summary:

The benefits of healthy eating for coronary heart disease can be achieved by:

- **Oily fish**: 2–4 times per week if you have had a heart attack and 1–2 times per week for everyone else. If you don't like eating the fish then consider omega-3 fish oil tablets
- **Fats** to be reduced generally in the diet and in particular to replace some saturated fats with monounsaturated fats
- **Fruit and vegetables**: eat five portions a day, with a good variety to provide appropriate vitamins, minerals, antioxidants and soluble fibre
- **Salt** to be reduced in the diet
- **Alcohol** to be consumed in moderation

In your handbook there is additional information on all of the things we have discussed today.

The figures quoted in this chapter are from British Cardiac Society et al. (2005) and National Institute for Clinical Excellence (2007).

Chapter 10

The Benefits of Regular Exercise and Making the Most of your Recovery (Week 6)

Session Plan for Week 6

1. The Benefits of Regular Exercise (15 minutes)
2. Exercise Practical (50 minutes)
   Tea and coffee break (10 minutes)
3. Making the Most of Your Recovery (45 minutes)

---

1. The Benefits of Regular Exercise

Aim of this talk: to highlight the wide range of benefits achieved by taking regular aerobic exercise.

*A great way to get this message across to the patient group is to represent the benefits pictorially and to get individuals to think about the different body systems that will benefit from regular exercise. Drawing a simple picture of the human body and asking the group to come up with benefits is one way of doing this. It is important to remind the group that these benefits will occur with **REGULAR** aerobic exercise and will only be maintained while the exercise is continued. It is also useful to remind the group that many of the benefits listed below take a considerable amount of time to build up and therefore will not necessarily be noticed immediately.*

Question to group: "What are the main benefits that you will get from regular aerobic exercise?"

Some of the main benefits from aerobic exercise are illustrated in Figure 10.1. The group may come up with others. It may be necessary to prompt an unresponsive group. Asking about the benefits of regular exercise to the Heart, or to the Body or to How you feel can be useful suggestions. Each benefit can be discussed in detail.

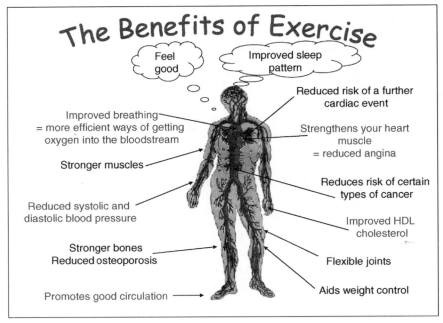

Figure 10.1 The benefits of exercise

So we have seen just how many benefits there are of regular exercise. Now we can start to put them into practice with today's exercise session!

2. Exercise Practical

Following the talk a practical exercise session is held using a circuit format to allow individuals of different abilities to work together.
Break for tea and coffee

3. Making the Most of Your Recovery

In this part of the session we are going to look at how we can make the most of our recovery following a cardiac event.
This section may appear lengthy as it covers a number of activities (e.g. driving, holidays, sexual activity) that the group may wish to return to following a cardiac event. Not all of these will necessarily be covered with every group.

We would hope that in time most people will get back to doing all of the activities that they were doing prior to their cardiac event. At this stage in time following your event, however, we would not necessarily expect you to be back doing all of those things. We know that for some people it can take up to a year or more to fully recover from a cardiac event both physically and psychologically. Others will already feel that they are back to "normal". We are all different, however, and we will want to get back to doing different things following a cardiac event. Some people may have had difficulties or complications and may be adjusting to a new "normality". One person's idea of what is normal will often differ from another's. Some people find that getting back to activities such as work, driving, sex and going on holiday can need a little thinking about, and it can take a while to regain a good level of confidence with regard to these activities.

Question to group: "Does anybody have any other activities that they may be concerned about getting back to?"
List responses on the whiteboard. Common examples are physical activities, gardening, sports, DIY, etc.

We mentioned that most people should be able to get back to doing all of the activities (and even more for some people!) that they were doing prior to their cardiac event. Others may not get back to doing some of their regular activities, and we will focus on some of the reasons why this can be. In particular we will look at the role that thoughts and feelings play, and how negative thinking specifically can affect our feelings and behaviours and result in some people not achieving the recovery that they may have hoped for.

Thoughts and Feelings

Draw the cognitive cycle of thoughts, feelings, behaviours and physical sensations on the whiteboard.
In Week 1 of the programme we talked about the impact that a cardiac event can have on an individual. We talked about how our thoughts, feelings and behaviours are all a normal part of everyday life, that they have an effect on each other and that the physical side of things can have an effect on us as well. We talked about how these thoughts, feelings and behaviours can result in positive cycles but can also result in vicious (or negative) cycles. In Week 1 we discussed how our interpretation of a particular physical sensation (a chest sensation) can be very different following a cardiac event and can potentially lead to a vicious

cycle of negative thoughts, feelings and behaviours. We discussed how before the cardiac event it would be likely that a chest sensation would be interpreted as indigestion and would result in taking an indigestion remedy. Following a cardiac event common thoughts such as "What if it's my heart . . .?" can lead to feelings of anxiety or worry and may result in behaviours such as taking GTN spray or phoning for an ambulance.

Anxiety

Negative thoughts can spring up at any point in the recovery process causing us to feel worried or anxious, but they are particularly common in the early stages of recovery. When we worry or are anxious, we start to expect the worst and to focus on all of the potential problems rather than taking a more realistic or balanced view of our situation. We think a lot of, "What if . . ." thoughts. Consider this example (*Draw the example given in Figure 10.2 on the whiteboard, starting with the negative thought.*)

The sequence of thoughts, feelings and behaviours in this example can become a damaging, vicious cycle. Over time, we could end up doing less and worrying more, possibly getting more symptoms and experiencing a worsening quality of life. We can also end up feeling fed up and low. Feeling fed up or low is common after a cardiac event, and patients can experience a variety of symptoms, including sadness, tearfulness, poor appetite, low motivation, lethargy

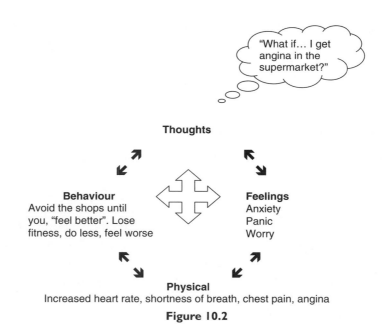

Figure 10.2

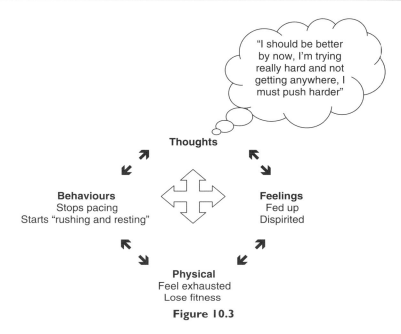

Figure 10.3

and sleep problems. When our spirits are low we tend to think more in terms of "Shoulds", "Musts" and "Nevers". We set ourselves unrealistic targets and "beat ourselves up" when we don't achieve them. For example, when we have been unwell or had a health event, we can often look to specific milestones to let us know if we think that we are making the recovery that we expected. We sometimes hear patients say things like "It's been six months since my heart attack. I *should* be feeling better by now. I'll *never* get back to my gardening." Having not been through this experience before, how can we possibly know that we should be better by this point in time? Yet we all tend to think in this way (*draw Figure 10.3 on the whiteboard*). This shows the effect these kind of thoughts can have on us.

If, for example, the worrying thought concerns getting angina in the super-market, then anxiety may be reduced by challenging the thought and replacing it with, "Angina will not damage my heart and will go away if I rest." Sometimes it can help to imagine what someone else might say or think in a situation, some-one that you find reassuring. The aim is not to stop having negative thoughts completely but to be less worried by them through this thought-challenging process. So rather than the vicious cycle that we saw in the diagram I've just drawn we might have a more positive cycle (*draw Figure 10.4*).

Similarly, challenging negative thoughts and replacing them with alterna-tives can help when you feel low or down.

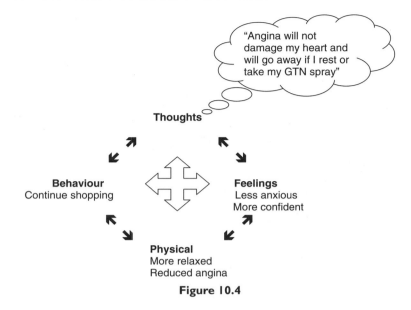

Figure 10.4

Remember that feeling down or low is common in the early stages of recovery, but these feelings tend to gradually lessen as time passes. Try and stay active, as exercise is a great "mood lifter", and make sure that you talk to people to let them know how you are feeling.

Hopefully we can all maintain positive cycles of thoughts, feelings and behaviours that will enable us to do all of the activities that we mentioned at the start of the session.

Driving

Question to group: "For those of you feeling a bit apprehensive about returning to driving, how could you start to pace yourself back into it?"

Usual responses include: "Start with shorter journeys at quieter times", "Have a passenger to begin with", "Work up to longer journeys", "Allow more comfort stops to keep you fresher", etc.

Keep an eye on your thinking and use the thought-challenging that we have discussed. Keep reassuring yourself mentally. For those of you not feeling anxious about driving, keep an eye on your concentration levels. You may find driving more tiring than usual at this stage of the recovery process, but we are not always aware of how tired we are behind the wheel. Allow more stops to keep you alert.

Physical Activities

Physical activities such as gardening, DIY, or sports, come down to good pacing. Build up to things gradually; watch out for arms up above your head for long periods, or thinking that you'll "just finish" an activity even though it will mean that you will be doing much more than you originally planned. Enlist help from others where necessary. You do not gain anything by being proud and pushing yourself too hard. Much of your recovery, in all areas of your life, can be managed by good pacing. Pacing is not just about fitness. If we feel a bit nervous or apprehensive about resuming some of our activities, work or hobbies, then using the pacing principles can help us to regain our confidence and move forward in a positive way with our lives.

Holidays

There is no reason why you should not enjoy a holiday after a cardiac event. However, going on holiday is an example of an activity that some people do not return to because of feelings of anxiety or lack of confidence. Typically people can have a number of negative thoughts about going on holiday and these thoughts can sometimes seem overwhelming (*draw Figure 10.5 on the whiteboard*).

   In this example a variety of negative thoughts have caused feelings of anxiety when left unchallenged, leading to one of two outcomes: either not going on holiday at all or going on holiday and feeling so stressed that you would probably not want to go again. The key to managing this situation is to plan well and challenge the negative thoughts:

- Make sure that you know where hospital and medical facilities are near where you are staying. This can be reassuring for some people.
- Divide medication into two, possibly by putting some into your main luggage and carrying another set with you. Also take extra amounts. This is a good strategy if you are worried about losing your medication. Taking a printed list of medication from your pharmacist will enable you to get replacement medication should you need to. Also check with NHS Direct regarding taking medications into your country of destination, as some countries will require a letter from your doctor. This will help you to avoid any unnecessary stress on arrival.
- There is no reason why you cannot fly after a cardiac event. If you are worried about a deep vein thrombosis (DVT) then it is suggested that you

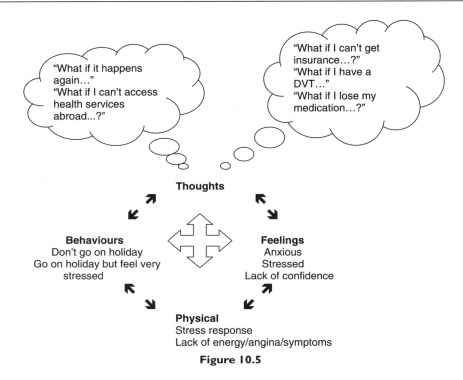

Figure 10.5

move around in your seat or cabin as much as possible, do leg exercises (which are often demonstrated on in-flight media), drink only water or soft drinks (avoiding alcohol) and take only short periods of sleep. This is the same advice that everyone should follow even if they have not had a cardiac event (and there is little extra risk for those who have had a cardiac event).

• It can be more difficult to get holiday insurance after a cardiac event, particularly in the first 12 months (and if you are waiting for an intervention), but most people should be able to get an acceptable quote if they put some time aside to shop around. The British Heart Foundation website provides useful information about holiday insurance.

The aim is to challenge negative thoughts (often in this case with good information) so that your confidence increases, you feel excited about going on holiday and you go and have a good time, so that when you return you begin planning to go again!

Remember the pacing principles as well. You may gain confidence to tackle longer journeys by having a short break first.

Sex

Research shows that up to half of cardiac patients do not resume their sex lives after their cardiac event. Some people are not concerned about this, but for others it is an important part of getting back to normal. There are a number of reasons why sexual difficulties can occur:

- Coronary heart disease
- Diabetes
- Medication
- Anxiety (either in yourself or your partner)

It is important that you are aware of these issues so that you can get advice and information if you are experiencing problems. Your GP can consider the issues relevant to you and may prescribe or change medications, or refer you on for specialist advice.

This is an area where vicious cycles can be common, often caused by worrying thoughts (*draw Figure 10.6 on the whiteboard*).

In Week 2 we described how the stress response was our life-saving response. When we get anxious, our body goes onto red alert, expecting something bad to happen, and all non-essential systems in the body are shut down in order to get blood to the big working muscles. The only response your body is preparing for is to fight something, to run away or to play dead and (hopefully!) our usual sex lives do not include these!

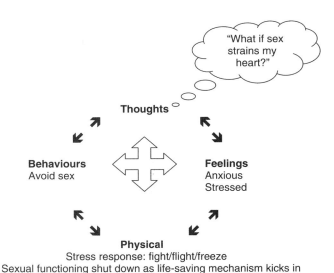

Figure 10.6

Anxiety alone can be enough to really interfere with your sexual functioning and that can be equally true of partners, if they have concerns about you overexerting yourself. This can have a huge impact on the quality of your relationship. Couples can stop holding hands or kissing and cuddling, in case it leads to sex. Some people can feel very demoralised if there are sexual problems. This is why it is important that anyone with concerns has a chat with their GP to see what can be done to help them.

From an exertion point of view, it can be reassuring for both you and your partner to know that the American College of Sports Medicine guidelines state that if you can manage a 20-minute walk on the flat and two flights of stairs, on a regular basis, with no symptoms, that is the usual level of exertion for most people's sex lives.

In summary:

- Learn to challenge your anxious or negative thoughts. Try to find an alternative perspective or viewpoint. This can be really powerful.
- Get support and make sure that you talk about your worries and concerns. Often, talking through worries helps us to get a better perspective on them and to feel reassured. Make use of friends and family, and your GP, practice nurse, and cardiac rehabilitation team.
- Get good, clear, accurate information about your health event, your risk factors and what you can do to manage them.
- Pace yourself. Return to your activities, hobbies, work, etc. in a gradual fashion if you are not feeling confident. Use the goal-setting principles we talked about in Week 1. You can pace yourself back to doing anything.
- Relaxation exercises are important to help reduce our stress levels and clear our thought processes.
- Exercise regularly to increase your confidence and fitness. Regular exercise helps us to cope with the constant demands of our everyday lives.

For further reading see Hawton et al. (2001).

Chapter 11

Staying Fit, Cardiac Medication and the Future! (Week 7)

Session Plan for Week 7

1. How to Stay Fit for Life (10 minutes)
2. Exercise Practical (50 minutes)
   Tea and coffee break (15 minutes)
3. Medication (35 minutes)
4. The Future! (10 minutes)

---

1. How to Stay Fit for Life

Aim of the talk: to equip patients with the knowledge of how to increase their exercise levels over time and to explore ideas of how to maintain exercise in the longer term.

The most important aspect of this talk is to remind individuals that in order to maintain all of the benefits of exercise (discussed in Week 6) exercise must be maintained for life.

How to Recognise that Your Exercise Levels Need to be Increased

When following an exercise programme over a period of time an individual should see an improvement in their exercise capacity. In order to challenge their body further their exercise prescription will need to be increased.

Question to group: "How might we know when our exercise level needs to be increased?"

Typical answers may include:

- *Our breathing rate has reduced (i.e. no longer getting slightly out of breath on exercising)*

- *A reduced score on the exercise scale (e.g. only scoring very light or light)*
- *Our heart rate is not getting into our training range.*

If any of the above answers apply then you can consider increasing the amount of exercise that you are doing!

The easiest way of explaining this to the group is to refer back to the FITT principle of exercise which was introduced in Week 1 of the programme. Figure 11.1 shows how this can be written on the whiteboard. The left-hand side of the shaded boxes refers to an example of a patient's current exercise level. The right-hand side of the boxes refers to an example of how each component of exercise can be increased.

When increasing our exercise level only one factor should be altered at a time. For example, if you are going to change the exercise frequency, no other changes to the exercise should be made (i.e. to the "intensity" of the exercise or "time" that you spend exercising). Ideally changes in exercise frequency and time should be made before considering any changes in exercise intensity. It is important to remember the principles of pacing, especially when starting a new exercise or activity.

Changing the **type** of exercise that you are doing will depend on individual preference. Walking is usually recommended in the early stages of recovery from a cardiac event. However, as time progresses you may wish to try alternative forms of aerobic exercise such as cycling or swimming.

Exercise classes (commonly using a circuit-training approach) and gym-based exercise programmes are also popular alternative options.

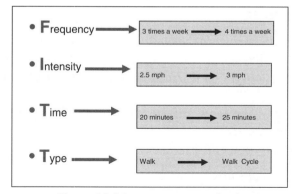

Figure 11.1 Increasing exercise levels

Dealing with Setbacks

When dealing with any sort of setback (e.g. further health problems, cold, flu, etc.) your exercise levels will need to be adjusted. For example, if you were to stop exercising for a few weeks because of a bad cold you will inevitably have lost some fitness by the time that you return to your exercise regime. It would therefore be advisable to reduce your level of exercise and gradually build it back up over a period of time.

Maintaining Exercise

Eventually you will reach a "plateau" with your exercise, whereby you are happy with the frequency and intensity of the exercise and the time that you spend exercising. At this stage it becomes a question of maintaining this level of exercise.

How to Keep Motivated to Exercise Regularly

Following the completion of a cardiac rehabilitation programme it is common for patients to experience a dip in their motivation levels. It is therefore important to consider ways in which you can remain motivated to exercise on a regular basis.

Question to group: "How can we keep our exercise going in the long term?"

The most common answers are presented in Figure 11.2. Write these on the whiteboard. This part of the session is a chance for patients and partners to help each other by sharing their ideas.

Setting Achievable Goals

The key to exercising successfully is to set goals that are both realistic and achievable for you. We have talked about setting achievable goals at different stages throughout the programme and it is vital that we keep this going in the future.

Developing a Routine

Having a routine can be important for some people in order to maintain their exercise. If it is in the diary or on the wall-planner that you are going for a walk

- Set achievable goals
- Get into a routine
- Find a type of exercise that is enjoyable
- Exercise with other people
- Join a Phase IV exercise class
- Have an indoor alternative when the weather is bad
- Reward yourself regularly
- Make it functional, e.g.
  - Walk to the paper shop
  - Walk the dog
  - Use the car less

Figure 11.2 Keeping your exercise going. . .

at a certain time and on a certain day of the week then it is more likely you will keep to it. Over time it becomes a habit, and it is therefore more likely that you will maintain it in the longer term.

Finding an Exercise that is Enjoyable

This is one of the key factors in keeping our exercise going in the long term. Both keeping variety in your exercise programme and finding a suitable type of exercise is vital. It can be helpful to make regular changes to your exercise programme, for example trying a different route when out walking.

Exercising with Other People

Exercising with other people can help in keeping up motivation levels. Making an agreement to meet a friend at a particular time of week in order to exercise can mean that you are more likely to engage in that behaviour. It can also mean that exercising can become a social occasion too!

Joining a Phase IV Exercise Class

Following completion of a Phase III cardiac rehabilitation programme many areas of the country now offer ongoing exercise sessions, or Phase IV classes. These tend to be run by local leisure centres or heart support groups and can provide you with ongoing exercise classes. The set-up of these sessions will vary from place to place, but normally they run as circuit-training classes or gym programmes. Some programmes will also cater for partners of CHD patients, allowing them to attend the exercise sessions as well.

Having an Indoor Alternative

Having a back-up plan for when the weather is bad can be useful. Many people find that during the winter months, when the weather is cold and wet, it is difficult to stay active. Having an alternative exercise to walking (for example going through a home exercise routine or going to an exercise class) can mean that your exercise is maintained regardless of the weather.

Giving out copies of the exercises used in the cardiac rehabilitation programme for patients to take home means they are able to run through an exercise routine in the comfort of their own home. This can be particularly useful for individuals who are less mobile or who are housebound.

Rewards

Reward yourself for good behaviour! For example, if you have been very good at keeping to your exercise routine for a month you might wish to arrange a nice meal out one evening to reward yourself! It doesn't matter what the reward is as long as you feel that you benefit from it.

Making Exercise Purposeful

Many of us find it hard to find the time to exercise so it can be important to try and fit exercise into our everyday lives—for example, walking to the paper shop rather than using the car if it is a short journey.

BACR Phase IV Exercise Instructor Courses

The British Association for Cardiac Rehabilitation Phase IV Exercise Instructor Training Programme (funded by the British Heart Foundation) was launched in 1997 to provide specialist training for exercise professionals who want to prescribe and deliver exercise programmes as part of the overall long-term management of individuals with heart disease. There are now almost 2,000 qualified instructors spread across the UK.

BACR is the national organisation for all professionals involved in the field of cardiac rehabilitation and is an affiliated group of the British Cardiovascular Society. BACR promotes good practice, produces national guidelines, and develops educational programmes within the field of cardiac rehabilitation.

The course runs nationwide and is open to experienced exercise professionals. The qualification attracts 20 REPS (Register of Exercise Professionals) points and requires revalidation every three years. For further details on the course please see the contact details below.

BACR Phase IV
Town Hall Exchange,
Castle Street,
Farnham,
Surrey,
GU9 7ND
Email info@bacrphaseiv.co.uk
Phone 01252 720640
Fax 01252 720601

2. Exercise Practical

Following the talk a practical exercise session is held using a circuit format to allow individuals of different abilities to work together.
Break for tea and coffee

3. Medication

In this final session we are going to discuss the medication that you are likely to be prescribed following a cardiac event. We will look at what these medications are, the reasons for taking them, what the medications do and the possible side-effects of taking them.

Secondary Prevention

Following a cardiac event you may be prescribed a number of different medications to reduce the risk of having another cardiac event. This is called *secondary prevention* medication and the reasons for taking it can differ to the reasons for taking the medication that you may have for other conditions. For example, if you have a chest infection you may have a temperature and productive cough and need to be prescribed antibiotics by your GP. Over the course of seven days your temperature settles and you no longer have the cough and you feel much better. When the course of treatment ends you will no longer need to take the antibiotics. In this situation you have felt better as a result of taking the antibiotics.

The secondary prevention medications differ, in that you may not feel any different while you are taking the medication. However, we know that these medications play a very important part in the management of your CHD.

Question to group: "Why do you need to take medication following a cardiac event?"
Acknowledge the groups answers where appropriate.

Cardiac medications work in a different way to (for instance) antibiotics, and their main purpose will be to **reduce the risk of you having a further cardiac event**. Because of this, some of the medications you will have been prescribed will need to be taken for the rest of your life. It is therefore important that in the future you do not become complacent and think it is OK to stop taking the medications, as you will only have the benefits for as long as you are taking them.

There are a number of different medications that you may be prescribed after a cardiac event (although not everybody will be prescribed all of the cardiac medications that we are going to discuss today). The medication that you are on will depend on what kind of cardiac event you have experienced and the views of your cardiologist regarding what is the best medication for you as an individual.

Question to group: "What medications might you be prescribed following a cardiac event?"
Answers may include a variety of different medications although the focus of this session will be specifically on the four main cardiac medications: anti-platelets, statins, beta-blockers and ACE-inhibitors. Write these medications on the whiteboard.
Other cardiac medications that the group mention can be explained at the end of the session.

The following format may be useful to use for each group of tablets (see Table 11.1).

First of all we are going to look at a group of tablets called the **anti-platelets**. This medication helps to make our blood less "sticky".

Table 11.1 Medications for coronary heart disease

To reduce the risk of a further cardiac event			
1. Anti-platelet			
2. Beta-blockers			
3. Cholesterol-lowering			
4. ACE-inhibitors			
Medication	**Dose**	**What it does**	**Other info./side-effects**
1. Anti-platelets e.g. Aspirin	75 mg	Reduces stickiness of blood	Do not take on empty stomach as can cause gastric irritation
		Helps to reduce risk of further cardiac event	May bruise more easily and bleed for longer

Anti-platelets

Everyone should be on an anti-platelet medication after having a cardiac event.

> **Question to group: "Which medications are you taking that 'thin' your blood?"**

Aspirin

Aspirin reduces the risk of a having a heart attack or angina and does this by reducing the stickiness of the blood. This then helps to prevent clots from occurring in the coronary arteries. Generally you would be prescribed a small dose of Aspirin (usually 75 mg, although you can be on a higher dose if it is deemed necessary). Aspirin should not be taken on an empty stomach as it can cause gastric irritation. Aspirin will be prescribed for the rest of your life unless you have any problems with taking it.

Clopidogrel

Clopidogrel can also be used to reduce the risk of a heart attack or angina and again will usually be prescribed in a 75 mg dose. If you cannot take Aspirin because it does not agree with you then Clopidogrel can be used instead. However, it is now common to be on both Aspirin and Clopidogrel after a heart attack for a period of time. You will certainly be on both of these medications if you have had a coronary stent inserted. In this instance Clopidogrel will help protect the stent from furring up and should be taken for one year. If you are taking two anti-platelets together (e.g. Aspirin and Clopidogrel) you may find that you bruise more easily, and if you cut yourself it is normal that you may bleed a little longer than previously.

Warfarin

For some people it will have been decided that Warfarin is the most appropriate drug. This can be for a number of reasons. It might be that you have a condition called *atrial fibrillation* (this is when your heart beats irregularly) or it may be that you have had surgery on a heart valve.

Beta-blockers

The second group of medications that you may be on are called **beta-blockers**.
    On the white board erase the information on anti-platelets and then use the table for the information on beta-blockers.

Question to group: "What are the names of the beta-blockers that you have been prescribed?"
Write the names on the whiteboard and put the information into the table as above for Aspirin.

Beta-blockers block the action of adrenaline, and by doing this they slow the heart rate and reduce the amount of work that the heart has to do. This in turn helps to reduce the symptoms of angina. Beta-blockers also help to reduce your blood pressure. There are a number of different beta-blockers that you may be prescribed.

The names of the beta-blockers tend to end in "-olol". Examples are Biso-prolol, Metoprolol and Atenolol. Not everyone will be on a beta-blocker after a cardiac event. However, if you have had a *heart attack* then the evidence suggests that you should be on a beta-blocker for up to one year following your heart attack. This is, therefore, one of the medications that might be stopped by your cardiologist. If, however, the beta-blocker is helping to control your blood pressure then it would usually be continued. Some people who have asthma or chest conditions may not be suitable for a beta-blocker.

A side-effect of beta-blockers in some people is cold hands and feet. Others can suffer from impotence or erectile dysfunction. If you think that you are having a side-effect from your beta-blocker then you do not need to suffer in silence; it is best to talk it through with your GP. There may be an alternative medication that will not give you the side-effect.

ACE-inhibitors

The next group of medications that we are going to discuss is called the **ACE-inhibitors**.

Question to group: "What are the names of the ACE-inhibitors that you have been prescribed? What do you think they do?"
Write the names on the whiteboard and add information to the table.

ACE-inhibitors help the arteries to relax and this has an effect on lowering the blood pressure and making it easier for the heart to pump more efficiently. Ace-inhibitors can also help to keep the heart muscle in good shape, which also helps it to pump more efficiently.

Common ACE-inhibitors are Ramipril, Captopril, Lisinopril or Perindopril. The names of the ACE-inhibitors tend to end in "-pril", but there is also another type of ACE-inhibitor (known as an ACE II), such as Valsartan or Candesartan, whose names end in "-tan".

Not everyone will be on an ACE-inhibitor, but if you are then you will normally be started off on a low dose (e.g. 2.5 mg of Ramipril). If a blood test shows that the medication has not affected your kidney functioning then generally the dose will be increased. This can seem a bit strange as previously you may have had the experience of a doctor telling you that you are doing well and so your medication can be reduced! With some of the cardiac medication it is different in that the evidence for its effective use comes from the evaluation of its use at a higher dose. That may be the dose that the doctor is aiming for.

A common side-effect of the ACE-inhibitors is a dry, tickly cough. If the cough is not too bothersome and is not unduly affecting your quality of life (for example it is not keeping you awake at night) then you may decide that it is worth putting up with. If it is a major problem for you, an ACE II medication (e.g. Valsartan, Candesartan) can be prescribed, and although they have the same benefits as an ACE-inhibitor they do not tend to carry the side-effect of a dry cough.

Statins

The final group of tablets that we are going to discuss and one that most of you will have been prescribed are called **statins**.

> **Question to group: "What are the names of the statins that you have been prescribed? What do you think they do?"**
> *Write the names on the whiteboard and add to the table.*

Statins are one of the medications that can be prescribed to reduce the level of cholesterol.

The common statins that you will be prescribed are Simvastatin, Atorvastatin or Rosuvastatin. Simvastatin is the most common statin and for most people a 40 mg dose of Simvastatin will reduce their total cholesterol level to below 4.0 or alternatively reduce it by 25 per cent. If this is not the case then it might be necessary to take either Atorvastatin or Rosuvastatin instead in order to achieve the target cholesterol level.

Statins work by lowering the amount of cholesterol produced by your liver. Some of the statins need to be taken at night to be most effective. It is also thought that statins help to stabilise the plaques in the arteries making them less likely to rupture.

The main side-effect of statins (although it is not a common side-effect) is problems with muscles, resulting in pain, tenderness or weakness. The pain will usually affect the major muscle groups such as the arms and the legs and can slowly get worse over time. If you experience unexplained muscle pain, tenderness or weakness then you would need to inform your GP. A blood test can distinguish whether this is a side-effect of the statin (which would be stopped if it was identified as such). It is possible that an alternative statin may then be prescribed that would not cause this side-effect. It is advised that you do not eat grapefruit or drink grapefruit juice if you are taking certain statins as it can interact with the medication, making the statin more potent.

Other cardiac medications can be briefly discussed at this point if necessary.

Reading the leaflet that comes with your medication can make you think that you are suffering from a number of the side-effects that are listed! Most people, though, will be able to take the cardiac medication with minimal or no side-effects at all. However, it is important not to ignore any new symptoms or side-effects of medication and to consult with your GP if you do suffer any new side-effects.

In summary:

- We take cardiac medication after a cardiac event to help reduce the risk of having another cardiac event (secondary prevention)
- The main groups of cardiac medication which reduce this risk are: anti-platelets, beta-blockers, ACE-inhibitors and statins

- You may not be on all of the main cardiac medications but your cardiologist will decide which medications are individually right for you
- If you experience any side-effects from your medication then discuss it with your GP. There may be an alternative that can be prescribed

Figures for cardiac medication have been taken from National Institute for Clinical Excellence (2007) and Department of Health and British Heart Foundation (2007b).

4. The Future!

First of all, congratulations for getting to the end of the cardiac rehabilitation programme. By attending cardiac rehabilitation you have made a major investment in your future health and done something very positive to reduce the chances of having another cardiac event. Well done!

Follow-up Sessions

Although we have now reached the end of the seven-week programme it is not quite the end of cardiac rehabilitation as we do have two follow-up sessions to come. The first of these sessions will be approximately eight to ten weeks from today. The second session will be approximately eight months from now, or six months after the first follow-up session. We will send you a letter with the date and time of the first follow-up and we will also send you another of our cardiac rehabilitation questionnaires to fill in and bring to the session. The information that we get from these questionnaires is invaluable both in helping us know how well you are doing as individuals and also whether we are making a difference to you as a group of patients by providing this service. So thank you in advance for bringing those with you to the follow-up.

The follow-up sessions will last for an hour and we will have an informal discussion on how things have been for you over the previous eight to ten weeks (or, at the second follow-up, six to eight months). It is our chance to reinforce some of the things that we have talked about on the programme (and that you may have forgotten in the intervening weeks!). It is also your chance to tell us about the things that have gone well for you or perhaps not so well, to tell us about any problems that you may have had and to ask any questions of the team.

It is common for some people to experience a dip in mood when they have completed a group programme such as cardiac rehabilitation. This is quite normal, and for most people this will pass within a week or two as you return to all of the things that you would normally be doing. If you do have some free time on the day that you have been attending cardiac rehabilitation then think about using it productively, maybe doing an extra session of aerobic exercise or using the time for yourself to do something that you enjoy or that helps you to relax.

Setbacks

Setbacks will naturally occur for some people and the important thing is that we treat then as exactly that, *setbacks*, rather than catastrophes! For some people it may be having a bad cold or the flu that sets them back. A common negative thought is, "I was doing so well and now this has put me right back to the beginning again." Challenge these thoughts, as most often they will not be true! More likely it will just take a little time to get back to where you were before your setback. At times like this it is crucial to remember the pacing principles that we have talked about throughout the programme. If you are unwell for any reason and you are not doing your normal activity or exercise then you will inevitably lose some fitness. The key is to come down a rung or two on the goal-setting ladder when you feel well enough to resume your activities. By reducing your baseline and doing a bit less than you were before you were unwell you will reduce the likelihood of overdoing it and getting into the cycle of "rushing and resting" that can be so problematic.

Planning, Pacing and Goal-setting

The most important thing to take away from the programme is that cardiac rehabilitation does not stop when the course stops. What is vital is what you do from now on for the rest of your life! Goal-setting and pacing continue to be crucially important into the future. If you are taking on new activities or making lifestyle changes then you need to plan what you want to achieve and how you are going to get there. Setting achievable goals, having a baseline and pacing ourselves towards our goals is the way forward with any new activity. Basing what we do on how we feel, getting into a cycle of good and bad days and "rushing and resting" is most definitely not! At the follow-up sessions it is generally those people who are pacing themselves well who are doing better and achieving more.

Hopefully from the course we have learned new skills and different ways of doing things. It is important to maintain any lifestyle changes that we have made for life. It is also important to remember that, if we are going to make changes in the future, they need to be made one at a time and they need to be realistic. Setting unachievable goals will result in failure. On the other hand, we need to reward ourselves for our achievements. Build in rewards so that you have good things to look forward to. It will help to maintain any lifestyle changes into the future. Now is a good time to take stock of your recovery so far and to think what realistic goals you might like to set yourself before you come back for our follow-up session.

Managing Stress

Stress management is a skill, and like any other skill it is one that we need to practise. The key to successfully coping with stress is to recognise what is causing it and to react early. If we feel we are getting stressed then we need to use it as a cue to relax. Use breaks in activity, for example sitting in the car in traffic or standing at a queue in the post office, to actively relax. Beforehand these might have been the times when our stress levels would be raised. Now they are an opportunity to practise relaxation. Similarly, when returning to work or getting back into any normal routine, plan in relaxation time. Get into the habit of doing a couple of abdominal breaths at regular times throughout the day. Instead of dashing to the phone, let it ring one more time and do an abdominal breath. Similarly, at every red traffic light make sure that you do a couple of abdominal breaths. Very quickly it will become part of your routine.

If things start getting on top of you remember the talk on *positive thinking*. Write down negative thoughts, or talk to someone about what is troubling you. If time pressure is the problem (i.e. there is not enough time for everything that you need to do) write everything down and prioritise your needs. Ask yourself, "What really needs to be done?" Look at what you can do differently. Ask yourself, "What can I change?" If the problems persist then please feel free to contact a member of the cardiac rehabilitation team. The handbook that we gave you in Week 1 of the programme has the telephone number of the cardiac rehabilitation office inside. If you have any questions or queries over the next eight to ten weeks then you are very welcome to give the office a call and we can discuss any issues that you may have. If we are not able to answer your question then we can normally find somebody who can!

And finally just to say well done again and keep up the good work! We will see you in eight to ten weeks' time for your first follow-up—and remember that your cardiac rehabilitation team is only a telephone call away.

Appendix 1: Assessment Documentation

Gloucestershire Hospitals *NHS*
NHS Foundation Trust

Gloucestershire Cardiac Rehabilitation Service
Assessment Document

Enter details or affix Hospital label here

Name	
Address	
Date of Birth	
Hospital No.	

Cardiac Rehabilitation No.		Home Phone Number	
Next of Kin		Telephone Number	
GP Practice		Telephone Number	

Admission Date		Discharge Date		Consultant	
Diagnosis					
Date of Operation					
Thrombolysis?		Streptokinase?		Card & Advice Given?	
Relevant History / Information					

ETT		Date		ECHO		Date	
ANGIO		Date		PCI		Date	

Post Surgical Assessment

Referred From			
Chest Discomfort		Wound Pain	
Thoracic Exercise		Analgesia discussed	
Physical Risk Assessment			
Physical Limitations			

Secondary Prevention Medication Prescribed (If no, explain why)

Aspirin	
Clopidogrel	
Beta Blocker	
Statin	
ACE Inhibitor	

Cardiac Rehabilitation Programme (Select Yes / No where appropriate)

Accepted a place on the Cardiac Rehabilitation programme.	
Preferred venue:	
Did not accept place because:	
Not offered a place because:	
Patient has contact number and can access the service at any time.	
Referrals made; (please specify)	

Information Given (Select Yes / No where appropriate)

Explained diagnosis		Information booklet given		Explained use of GTN & when	
Explained what angina is		Patient has GTN prescribed		to call for help	

Signature		Print Name	
Designation		Date	

To be filed in the other professional records that are not incuded in the clinical records section of the Health Record

Name			Hospital No.		

Risk Factor	Assessment			Action / Advice	(Select Yes / No where appropriate)	
Smoking	Ex-smoker?		Non-smoker?		Referred to Smoking Cessation Team	
	Smoker?		per day			
Blood Pressure	High blood pressure			Advised to aim for BP<		
				Specific advice for Diabetes		
Cholesterol	Date			Statin prescribed		
	Total Cholesterol		mmol / L	Advised to have fasting cholesterol checked		
				in 3 months		
				Advised to aim for total cholesterol < 4mmol/L or reduce total by 25% whichever is the lowest figure.		
Family history	Family history?					
Obesity	BMI > 30?					
Prolonged stress	Prolonged stress					
Lack of exercise	Lack of exercise			Pacing explained		
				Aerobic excercise explained		
Excess alcohol	Excess alcohol			Advised upper level of safe drinking		
	Average units per day			Men - 3 units per day		
				Women - 2 units per day		
Diabetes	Diabetes					
	Type			Advised needs to be reviewed in 3 months?		
	Control			Commenced Insulin		

Lifestyle Factors						
Occupation	Job				Hours / week	
					Medical Sick Certificate issued for	weeks
Driving	Driving licence type				Advised must not drive for	weeks
				Advised to inform insurance company		
Sexual activity	Discussed					
Hobbies						
Diet	Advised to eat 1-2 portions of oily fish per week or take fish oil capsules					
	Advised to eat 2-3 portions of oily fish per week or take fish oil capsules					
	Advised to eat 5 portions of fruit & vegetables per day					
	Advised to reduce saturated fat and choose monounsaturated fats					

Other relevant information		

Signature		Print Name	
Designation		Date	

This is not a Discharge Summary. All details correct at the time of assessment.

Cardiac Rehabilitation Offices:
Gloucestershire Royal Hospital 08454 228278 - Cheltenham General Hospital 08454 223535

Page 2

Appendix 2: Letter of Invitation

Gloucestershire Hospitals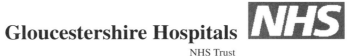

NHS Trust

All correspondence and enquires to:

Cardiac Rehabilitation Office
Cheltenham General Hospital
St Lukes Wing
Sandford Road
Cheltenham GL53 7AN
08454 223535

Patient name and address

Date: 2nd September 2008

Dear

A place has been booked for you on the Cardiac Rehabilitation Programme:

Where: **St Pauls Medical Centre, Physiotherapy Department (The Old Chapel) 121 Swindon Road, Cheltenham GL50 4DP**

Date: **Wednesday 10th September 2008**

Time: **1.30pm to 3.30pm**

Then every Wednesday for a total of seven weeks. Each session is two hours long and it is recommended that you attend all seven weeks of the programme. If you think that this will not be possible please telephone on the above number for advice.

Who/What to bring:

You are welcome to bring your partner or a friend with you. Please complete the enclosed questionnaire and bring it with you to the first session. As the programme includes an exercise component we recommend that you wear flat, comfortable shoes and comfortable clothing from Week 2. We do not exercise on Week 1.

Why attend?

Attending a cardiac rehabilitation programme is a proven way to ensure the best possible recovery for yourself. By attending, you will be following the current medical and nursing guidelines and recommendations. Also, during the programme, the specialist team will be on hand to give you advice, support and information to help you make informed choices about your rehabilitation.

To accept, cancel or request an alternative date:

Please return the enclosed pink reply slip as soon as possible as places are very limited and would need to be reallocated to enable us to run the service efficiently.

Yours sincerely

The Cardiac Rehabilitation Team
Chair:
Dame Janet Trotter DBE

Chief Executive:
Dr Frank Harsent
Phd MBA

References

Bath, J.P., Giles, M., Harrison, J., Anderson, A., Gallacher, M., Callen, S. and Earll, L. (2004) Reporting the NSF targets for cardiac rehabilitation in Gloucestershire. *European Journal of Cardiovascular Prevention and Rehabilitation*, 11 (suppl. 1).

Beswick, A., Rees, K., Griebsch, I., Taylor, F., Burke, M., West, R., Victory, J., Brown, J., Taylor, R. and Ebrahim, S. (2004) Provision, uptake and cost of cardiac rehabilitation programmes: improving services to under-represented groups. *Health Technology Assessment*, 8, 41.

Bethell, H., Evans, J., Turner, S. and Lewin, R. (2007) The rise and fall of cardiac rehabilitation in the United Kingdom since1998. *Journal of Public Health*, 29(1), 57–61.

Bethell, H., Turner, S., Evans, J. and Rose, L. (2001) Cardiac rehabilitation in the United Kingdom: how complete is the provision? *Journal of Cardiopulmonary Rehabilitation*, 21(2), 111–115.

Borg, G. (1998) *Borg's Perceived Exertion and Pain Scales*. Stockholm: Human Kinetics.

Brodie, D., Bethell, H. and Breen, S. (2006) Cardiac rehabilitation in England: a detailed national survey. *European Journal of Cardiovascular Prevention and Rehabilitation*, 13(1), 122–128.

British Association for Cardiac Rehabilitation (2006) *British Association for Cardiac Rehabilitation Training Module*. Leeds: Human Kinetics.

British Association for Cardiac Rehabilitation (2007) *British Association for Cardiac Rehabilitation Standards and Core Components for Cardiac Rehabilitation*. BACR.

British Cardiac Society, British Hypertension Society, Diabetes UK, Heart UK, Primary Care Cardiovascular Society and the Stroke Association (2005) Joint British Societies Guidelines on Prevention of Cardiovascular Disease in Clinical Practice. *Heart*, 91, 1–52.

British Heart Foundation (2004) *Stress and your Heart*. London: BHF.

British Heart Foundation (2006) *Heart Information Series No. 6: Angina*. London: BHF.

British Heart Foundation (2007a) Factfile No. 5: Ethnic Differences in Cardiovascular Risk. London: BHF.

British Heart Foundation (2007b) *Heart Information Series No. 3: Reducing Your Blood Cholesterol*. London: BHF.

British Heart Foundation (2008) Heartstats. www.heartstats.org.

Broadbent, E., Petrie, K., Main, J. and Weinman, J. (2006) The Brief Illness Perception Questionnaire. *Journal of Psychosomatic Research*, 60(6), 631–637.

Bunker, S.J ., Colquhoun, D.M., Esler, M.D., Hickie, I.B., Hunt, D., Jelinek, V.M., Oldenburg, B.F., Peach, H.G., Ruth, D., Tennant, C.C. and Tonkin, A.M. (2003) Position Statement. "Stress" and coronary heart disease: psychosocial risk factors. *Medical Journal of Australia*, 178(6), 272–276.

Cardiac Rehabilitation Gloucestershire (2004) *Annual Report: 2003–2004 Cardiac Rehabilitation*. Gloucester: Gloucestershire Hospitals NHS Trust.

Clark, A., Hartling, L., Vandermeer, B. and McAlister, F.A. (2005) Meta-analysis: secondary prevention programs for patients with coronary artery disease. *Annals of Internal Medicine*, 143(9), 659–672.

Dalal, H., Evans, P. and Campbell, J. (2004) Recent developments in secondary prevention and cardiac rehabilitation after acute myocardial infarction. *British Medical Journal*, 328, 693–697.

Daly, J., Sindone, A., Thompson, D., Hancock, K., Chang, E. and Davidson, P. (2002) Barriers to participation in and adherence to cardiac rehabilitation programs: a critical literature review. *Progress in Cardiovascular Nursing*, 17(1), 8–17.

Department of Health (2000) *National Service Framework for Coronary Heart Disease*. London: Department of Health Publications.

Department of Health (2005) *Coronary Heart Disease*. London: Department of Health Publications.

Duits, A., Boeke, H., Duivenvoorden, H.J. and Passchier, J. (1996) Depression in patients undergoing cardiac surgery: a comment. *British Journal of Health Psychology*, 1, 283–286.

Dusseldorp, E., Van Elderen, T., Maes, S., Meulman, J. and Kraaij, V. (1999) A meta-analysis of psycho-educational programs for coronary heart disease patients. *Health Psychology*, 18(5), 506–519.

Engblom, E., Ronnemaa, T., Hamalainen, H., Kallio, V., Vanttinen, E. and Knuts, L.R. (1992) Coronary heart disease risk factors before and after bypass surgery: results of a controlled trial on multi-factorial rehabilitation. *European Heart Journal*, 13, 232–237.

Fortune, D.G., Richards, H.L., Main, C.J. and Griffiths, C.E.M. (2000) Pathological worrying, illness perceptions and disease severity in patients with psoriasis. *British Journal of Health Psychology*, 5, 71–82.

Franklin, B., Bonzheim, K. and Timmis, G. (1998) Safety of medically supervised cardiac rehabilitation exercise therapy: a 16-year follow-up. *Chest*, 114, 902–906.

Frasure-Smith, N., Lesperance, F. and Talajic, M. (1993) Depression following myocardial infarction: impact on 6-month survival. *JAMA*, 270, 1819–1825.

Frasure-Smith, N., Lesperance, F. and Talajic, M. (1995) Depression and 18-month prognosis after myocardial infarction. *Circulation*, 91(4), 999–1005.

Hawton, K., Salkovskis, P., Kirk, J. and Clark, D. (2001) *Cognitive Behaviour Therapy for Psychiatric Problems: A Practical Guide*. Oxford: Oxford Medical Publications.

Herlitz, J., Wiklund, I., Caidahl, K., Karlson, B.W., Sjoland, H., Hartford, M., Haglid, M. and Karlson, T. (1999) Determinants of an impaired quality of life five years after coronary artery bypass surgery. *Heart*, 81, 342–346.

Jenkinson, C. and Layte, R. (1997) Development and testing of the UK SF-12. *Journal of Health Services Research Policy*, 2(1), 14–18.

Kugler, J., Seelbach, H. and Kruskemper, G.M. (1994) Effects of rehabilitation exercise programmes on anxiety and depression in coronary patients: a meta-analysis. *British Journal of Clinical Psychology*, 33(3), 401–410.

Lane, D., Carroll, D., Ring, C., Beevers, G. and Lip, G. (2002) The prevalence and persistence of depression and anxiety following myocardial infarction. *British Journal of Health Psychology*, 7, 11–21.

Leventhal, H. and Nerenz, D. (1985) The assessment of illness cognition. In Karoly, P. (ed.), *Measurement Strategies in Health Psychology*. New York: John Wiley: 517–554.

Leventhal, H., Meyer, D. and Nerenz, D. (1980) The common sense representation of illness danger. In Rachman, S. (ed.), *Medical Psychology*, 2, 7–30.

Lewin, B., Cay, E.L., Todd, I., Soryal, I., Goodfield, N., Bloomfield, P. and Elton, R. (1995) The Angina Management Programme: a rehabilitation treatment. *British Journal of Cardiology*, 2, 221–226.

Lewin, R., Ingleton, R., Newens, A. and Thompson, D. (1998) Adherence to cardiac rehabilitation guidelines: a survey of cardiac rehabilitation programmes in the United Kingdom. *British Medical Journal*, 316, 1354–1355.

Linden, W., Phillips, M.J. and Leclerc, J. (2007) Psychological treatment of cardiac patients: a meta-analysis. *European Heart Journal*, 28, 2972–2984.

Mayou, R. (1992) Clinical significance of research on quality of life after coronary artery surgery. In Walter, P.J. (ed.), *Quality of Life after Open Heart Surgery*. Dordrecht: Kluwer Academic: 185–192.

Mayou, R., Gill, D., Thompson, D., Day, A., Hicks, N., Volmink, J. and Neil, A. (2000) Depression and anxiety as predictors of outcome after myocardial infarction. *Psychosomatic Medicine*, 62, 212–219.

Michie, S., O'Connor, D., Bath, J., Giles, M. and Earll, L. (2005) Cardiac rehabilitation: the psychological changes that predict health outcome and healthy behaviour. *Psychology, Health and Medicine*, 10(1), 88–95.

Milani, R.V., Lavie, C.J. and Cassidy, M.M. (1996) Effects of cardiac rehabilitation and exercise training programs on depression in patients after major coronary events. *American Heart Journal*, 132(4), 726–731.

Moss-Morris, R. (1997) The role of illness cognitions and coping in the aetiology and maintenance of Chronic Fatigue Syndrome. In Petrie, K.J. and Weinman, J. (eds), *Perceptions of Health and Illness*. Amsterdam: Harwood Academic Press.

Murphy, B., Elliott, P., Higgins, R., Le Grande, M., Worcester, M., Goble, A. and Tatoulis, J. (2008) Anxiety and depression after coronary artery bypass graft surgery: most get better, some get worse. *European Journal of Cardiovascular Prevention and Rehabilitation*, 15(4), 434–440.

Murphy, H., Dickens, C., Creed, F. and Bernstein, R. (1999) Depression, illness perception and coping in rheumatoid arthritis. *Journal of Psychosomatic Research*, 46, 155–164.

National Iinstitute for Clinical Excellence (NICE) (2007) *Clinical Guidelines 48: Secondary Prevention in Primary and Secondary Care for Patients Following a Myocardial Infarction*. London: Department of Health.

O'Connor, G.T., Buring, J.E., Yusuf, S., Goldhaber, S.Z., Olmstead, E.M., Paffenbarger, R.S. and Hennekens, C.H. (1989) An overview of randomised trials of rehabilitation with exercise after myocardial infarction. *Circulation*, 82, 234–244.

Ogden, J. (2007) *Health Psychology: A Textbook* (4th edn). Milton Keynes: Open University Press.

Oldridge, N.B., Guyatt, G.H., Fischer, M.E. and Rimm, A.A. (1988) Cardiac rehabilitation after myocardial infarction: combined experience of randomised clinical trials. *Journal of the American Medical Association*, 260, 945–995.

Pell, J. (1997) Cardiac rehabilitation: a review of its effectiveness. *Coronary Health Care*, 1, 8–17.

Petrie, K., Cameron, L., Ellis, C., Buick, D. and Weinman, J. (2002) Changing illness perceptions after myocardial infarction: an early intervention randomized controlled trial. *Psychosomatic Medicine*, 64, 580–586.

Petrie, K., Weinman, J., Sharpe, N. and Buckley, J. (1996) Role of patients' view of their illness in predicting return to work and functioning after myocardial infarction: longitudinal study. *British Medical Journal*, 312, 1191–1194.

Scheinowitz, M. and Harpaz, D. (2005) Safety of cardiac rehabilitation in a medically supervised community-based programme. *Cardiology*, 103(3), 113–117.

Scottish Intercollegiate Guideline Network (2002) *Cardiac Rehabilitation: A National Clinical Guideline*. Edinburgh: Royal College of Physicians.

Seki, E., Watanabe, Y., Sunayama, S., Iwama, Y., Shimada, K. and Kawakami, K. (2003) Effects of Phase III cardiac rehabilitation programs on health-related quality of life in elderly patients with coronary heart disease. *Circulation*, 67, 73–77.

Stagmo, M., Westin, L., Carlsson, R. and Israelsson, B. (2001) Long-term effects on cholesterol levels and the utilization of lipid-lowering drugs of a hospital-based programme for secondary prevention of coronary artery disease. *Journal of Cardiovascular Risk*, 8, 243–248.

Stengrevics, S., Sirois, C., Schwartz, C., Friedman, R. and Domar, A. (1996) The prediction of cardiac surgery outcome based upon preoperative psychological factors. *Psychology and Health*, 11(4), 471–477.

Sundin, O., Lisspers, J., Hofman-Bang, C., Nygren, A., Ryden, L. and Ohaman, A. (2003) Comparing multi-factorial lifestyle interventions and stress management in coronary risk reduction. *International Journal of Behavioural Medicine*, 10, 191–204.

Taylor, R., Brown, A., Ebrahim, S., Jolliffe, J., Noorani, H., Rees, K., Skidmore, B., Stone, J., Thompson, D. and Oldridge, N. (2004) Exercise-based rehabilitation for patients with coronary heart disease: systematic review and meta-analysis of randomised controlled trials. *American Journal of Medicine*, 116, 682–692.

Thompson, D. and De Bono, D. (1999) How valuable is cardiac rehabilitation and who should get it? *Heart*, 82, 545–546.

Turk, D.C., Okifuji, A. and Scharff, L. (1995) Chronic pain and depression: role of perceived impact and perceived control in different age cohorts. *Pain*, 61, 93–101.

Turner, S., Bethell, H., Evans, J., Goddard, J. and Mullee, M. (2002) Patient characteristics and outcomes of cardiac rehabilitation. *Journal of Cardiopulmonary Rehabilitation*, 22(4), 253–260.

University of York, NHS Centre for Reviews and Dissemination (1998) Cardiac rehabilitation. *Effective Health Care*, 4(4), 1–12.

Vestold Heartcare Study (2003) Influence on lifestyle measures and five-year coronary risk by a comprehensive lifestyle intervention programme in patients with coronary heart disease. *European Journal of Cardiovascular Prevention and Rehabilitation*, 10, 429–437.

Walker, J. (2001) *Control and the Psychology of Health: Theory, Measurement and Applications*. Milton Keynes: Open University Press.

Wallston, K.A., Wallston, B.S., Smith, S. and Dobbins, C.J. (1987) Perceived control and health. *Current Psychology-Research and Reviews*, 6(1), 5–25.

Ware, J.E., Kosinski, M. and Keller, S.D. (1996) SF-12: an even shorter health survey. *Medical Outcomes Trust Bulletin*, 4, 2.

Weinman, J., Petrie, K., Moss-Morris, R. and Horne, R. (1996) The illness perception questionnaire: a new method for assessing the cognitive representation of illness. *Psychology and Health*, 11, 431–445.

West, R. (2002) *Rehabilitation after Myocardial Infarction: Multicentre Randomised Controlled Trial*. London: Department of Health Publications.

White, C.A. (2001) *Cognitive Behaviour Therapy for Chronic Medical Problems: A Guide to Assesment and Treatment in Practice*. Chichester: John Wiley.

Whitmarsh, A., Koutantji, M. and Sidell, K. (2003) Illness perceptions, mood and coping in predicting attendance at cardiac rehabilitation. *British Journal of Health Psychology*, 8, 209–221.

WHO Committee Report (1993) Rehabilitation after cardiovascular diseases, with special emphasis on developing countries. *World Health Organization Technical Report Series*, 831, 1–122.

Williams, B., Poulter, N.R. and Brown, M.S. (2004) British Hypertension Society guidelines for management of hypertension: report of the 4th working party of the BHS. *Journal of Human Hypertension*, 18, 139–185.

Williams, M. (2001) Exercise testing in cardiac rehabilitation: exercise prescription and beyond. *Cardiology Clinics*, 19(3), 414–431.

Williams, M. and Balady, G. (1999) *Guidelines for Cardiac Rehabilitation and Secondary Prevention Programs*. Champaign: Human Kinetics.

Wyer, S., Joseph, S. and Earl, L. (2001) Predicting attendance at cardiac rehabilitation: a review and recommendations. *Coronary Health Care*, 5(4), 171–177.

Zigmond, A.S. and Snaith, R.P. (1983) The Hospital Anxiety and Depression Scale. *Acta Psychiatrica Scandinavica*, 67, 361–370.

Index

Note: Abbreviations used: CHD for coronary heart disease; CR for cardiac rehabilitation